LESSONS *from a* COMPLEX CHILD

One Family's Journey Untangling the Mysteries
of Regression, Diagnosis, and Recovery

ELLEN WOODBRIAR

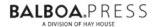
BALBOA.PRESS
A DIVISION OF HAY HOUSE

Balboa Press books may be ordered through booksellers or by contacting:

Balboa Press
A Division of Hay House
1663 Liberty Drive
Bloomington, IN 47403
www.balboapress.com
844-682-1282

Print information available on the last page.

ISBN: 978-1-9822-5498-8 (sc)
ISBN: 978-1-9822-5500-8 (hc)
ISBN: 978-1-9822-5499-5 (e)

Library of Congress Control Number: 2020917381

Balboa Press rev. date: 09/21/2020

This is a powerful book about a family's coping with a child's terrifying developmental regression and life-threatening illness – and their unending attempts to find help for him. Ms. Woodbriar writes in a warm, open, and vulnerable manner that lets us into her child's world – and to her own. Parents will be inspired and encouraged by her discussion of the emotional challenges experienced by everyone in a family with a medically complex child, including siblings. They will also benefit from her insights into a wide range of practical issues, including securing an appropriate school placement, finding a team of professionals who "get" your child, and dealing with insurance companies. Perhaps most importantly, this book will inspire parents to trust their own gut about what's right for their child - and to persevere in their search for ways to maximize their child's potential.

—**William R. Stixrud**, Ph.D.
Clinical Neuropsychologist and co-author of
The Self-Driven Child

This book gives the reader an intimate look inside a mother's experience of losing and finding her son due to complex medical issues. Ellen provides in-depth resources, insights, and her personal experience navigating the confusing mystery of Jackson's illness. She presents her journey through the heart of a mother and the mind of a clear-eyed professional.

—**Jennifer Asdorian**, M.S.,
Certificate of Clinical Competence (CCC)
-SpeechLanguage Pathologist (SPL)

Ms. Woodbriar's story about her family's journey to find answers and take steps toward healing her son gives families not just a 'how to' but also hope. She tells it with the passion she experienced as if every day she relives is like yesterday. For families who are embarking and going through discovery to understand their child's diagnosis, this story lays a groundwork for how to work with professionals as part of a team for a unified understanding, while setting goals and taking steps to achieve them!

—Suzanne Keith Blattner Ed.S.
Owner, Suzanne Keith Blattner and Associates
Educational Consultation and Advocacy
Kensington, Maryland

With the terror of her child's developmental regression, Ellen Woodbriar took on one of the most challenging conditions a parent can face - the complexity of a medical conundrum. She accomplished this by educating herself, relentless advocating, and seeking those practitioners who are literate in the multi-faceted puzzle that includes autism. With intuition and determination, she adjusted therapies based upon Jackson's progress and advice of a cadre of practitioners. This is the story of a mother's dedicated journey to secure the best and most successful treatments for her son.

—Dana Godbout Laake, RDH, MS, LDN
Licensed Dietitian Nutritionist
Dana Laake Nutrition
Co-author of The Kid-Friendly ADHD & Autism Cookbook
and The ADHD and Autism Nutritional Supplement Handbook.
Host of The Essentials of Healthy Living radio show.

A story of courage, resilience, persistence, patience, and the love of a mother to find an answer to what at first seemed to be an unsolvable challenge for her, her family, and her son. An inside look at a real and awe-inspiring journey: the work, dedication, and sacrifice, as well as the people and resources required to help her find the answers and provide the support necessary to move her child towards the independent young man that he is becoming today. For those of us, who are members of the "care community," a reminder to question what we think we know, keep our minds active, listen to our client's/patient's own wisdom, and keep our hearts open to helping those we support achieve what many think is impossible or improbable. A testament to the resilience in each of us, when we take the time to truly understand the nature of an other's distress rather than "treat" the symptoms of distress. A must read for all of us in the mental health field who work with kids and their families.

—**R. Patrick Savage**, Jr., Ph.D., Licensed Psychologist, and owner of R. Patrick Savage, Jr., Ph.D. & Associates, Olney and North Bethesda, Maryland.

This is a story of empowerment -- to learn to trust our intuition, to be an advocate, and to not be afraid to change course. Jackson's developmental journey started out smoothly with the typical colds and viruses all toddlers get, but by 30 months and multiple illnesses and rounds of antibiotics he regressed in language and motor skill with no clear-cut medical answer. Ellen Woodbriar shares this endearing and engaging story of encouragement, trust, determination and resiliency that made the difference between regression and recovery. This is a must read for parents, educators, pediatricians, and therapists.

—**Christine Sproat**, M.S., Occupational Therapist, and Director of Canyon Kids Pediatric Occupational Therapy Services, Bethesda, MD

For Jackson and Abby,
who taught me the meaning of unconditional love,
and
for all parents, caregivers, physicians, therapists,
and educators who dedicate their lives
to help children reach their fullest potential.

All disease begins in the gut.

—Hippocrates

ABOUT THE AUTHOR

• • • • • • • • • • •

Ellen Woodbriar is a dedicated mother, wife, sister, and friend. As a program manager, she spent most of her professional career helping organizations through transformational change. Personal experiences with her family, friends, and close colleagues led her through her own transformation resulting in this book, retirement from corporate life, more time with her family, and a career in life coaching.

If you are dealing with a medically complex situation and exploring diagnosis, please visit the Facebook page, Lessons from a Complex Child. Ellen has established this page for families like ours to share our stories, benefit from each other's knowledge, and feel supported in our journeys. We are not alone. You may also contact Ellen directly through e-mail at Ellen.Woodbriar@gmail.com.

CONTENTS

. . . .

ACKNOWLEDGMENTS

· · · · · · · · · · ·

Although it felt like it at times, this journey was not one William and I traveled alone. Many important and talented friends, family members, and professionals have helped, carefully guided, and in some instances led our family along our path. I introduce them throughout this book in the order in which our story unfolded.

By the time Jackson was in fifth grade, we had worked with one pediatric practice, two neurologists, two developmental pediatricians, one endocrinologist, one allergist, ten speech pathologists, seven occupational therapists, seven special educators, one special education advocate and consultant, one nutritionist, two neuropsychologists, one acupuncturist, one energy therapist, eight classroom teachers, and two Episcopal priests.

I will be indebted forever to these amazing people who dedicate their lives to caring for us and our children. Almost every one of them has worked diligently and tirelessly to help recover Jackson, but no one has worked as hard as Jackson.

This book would never have come to fruition without the help of many. I start with my reading buddies, Jennifer Asdorian, Sally Baldwin, and Judy Donohue; I would not have made it past the introduction without their encouragement. I'd also like to thank Mary Hornish for keeping my energy flowing, helping me stay grounded, and providing light and love throughout this writing and publishing process. I cherish these women's friendships and support and have nothing but gratitude for the time and effort they put in to helping tell this story.

Esther Goldenberg is a dedicated book coach with enviable patience. I will always be grateful to her for her support and expert guidance. Given the challenge of trying to reach multiple audiences with varying skill sets (therapists, teachers, physicians, parents), this book has been through an extensive editing process. I humbly thank Judy Donohue and Esther Goldenberg (again); Kate Green; Ulrike Guthrie; Dana Laake RDH, MS, LDN; Mary Riley, Peggy Riley; Ann Roberts, MD; John Tyler; Sara Wildberger; and Mary Oxley and the other staff at Balboa Press who contributed to this publication. They will never know how much I appreciate the time and talent they have dedicated to this project.

I respectfully thank Jackson and Abby for letting me tell our story in the hopes of helping so many others. Most importantly, I thank William, my husband, the father of my children, my love, and my best friend, for partnering with me as we untangled the mysteries of a medically complex child.

INTRODUCTION

. . . .

I write this book to tell you our story, a story of a journey with a healthy beginning, frightening middle, and a fortunate outcome.

At twenty-nine months, my son, Jackson, had met all his developmental milestones. He spoke in full sentences, knew his ABCs and colors, had well-developed fine and gross motor skills, was affectionate, had perfect eye contact, loved to talk, and was extremely social.

Six months later, just after Jackson's third birthday, neurologists couldn't rule out that he might have a malignant form of epilepsy, some form of neurodegenerative disorder, have regressive encephalopathy, be autistic, or have a pervasive developmental disorder (PDD).

What could possibly have caused the regression he experienced over a four-month period, the irritability he was exhibiting, the sixty to eighty seizures he was enduring each day, and the autistic-like behaviors he had developed?

I have always believed in functional medicine: understanding all variables contributing to a medical problem and not treating symptoms alone. If we started out by treating Jackson's symptoms, how would we know that we were solving the underlying problem? Although I understand that some disorders can present for the first time at the two- to three-year mark, autism spectrum disorders (ASD) or autistic-like symptoms are typically observed before twenty-nine months. Perhaps there was more depth to Jackson's symptoms than was obvious?

Although I'm not a physician and don't work in the health care profession, I have lived through the regression and recovery of my own child. This experience has led me to form the opinion that, potentially, too many children are being put on the autism spectrum. Some children, like Jackson, with ASD-like symptoms are not autistic and therefore are not receiving the full breadth of intervention that could potentially help them recover. Do I have proof of this? No, because from my experience, and up until this point, there has not been enough research, that the medical profession recognizes as reliable, made available to the public or to parents like me to identify the root cause of some symptoms.

Information is, however, starting to emerge, in books such as *Changing the Course of Autism: A Scientific Approach for Parents and Physicians; Bugs, Bowels, and Behavior; Is It Leaky Gut or Leaky Gut Syndrome?;* and *The Myth of Autism.* My perspective comes from my experience with my own child. I feel a compelling sense of responsibility to share that experience with others who are also searching for the right diagnosis for a child's symptoms.

The purpose of my telling this story is not to give anyone or any family false hope but, with good reason, to encourage you to leave no stone unturned in treating a medically complex child. It takes passionate determination and tenacity to find underlying and seemingly hidden causes of complex illnesses and to see the journey through to recovery when possible.

I tell Jackson's story:

First, because I believe in a parent's intuition. In the absence of a clear and compelling answer, it is important to question any diagnosis given to your child. Parents of a child with complex medical concerns have to find the stamina, intelligence, faith, and assertiveness to partner with medical professionals and other experts, without surrendering their own accountability and insight into their child's development.

Second, because as a parent or legal guardian, you are the most important advocate your child will ever have. No one else will love your child, ache for your child, or fight for your child the way you would. Regardless of your child's particular needs, most other people won't ever see him or her as the perfect and divine little soul that you see. You do not have to settle for any service, service provider, or advice that you believe does not have your child's best interest at heart. Learn from the less than optimal experiences and move on.

Third, because I hope to encourage even one other parent, physician, teacher, or therapist to look beyond the obvious and dig as deeply as necessary to help recover a child. I hope Jackson's story and the information in this book will offer a new and enlightening perspective to parents and to those who work with, but have not raised, a medically complex child. The first rule is to do no harm to a child; the second is to be open to new research and alternative therapies. We have a public health crisis on our hands; common sense tells us that what we've always done isn't working anymore.

Finally, because I want to validate for parents and caregivers that many paths in helping a medically complicated child recover or redevelop are long and seemingly blazed alone. Knowing that you are not alone and that others—myself included—have navigated similar paths before you can help mitigate what otherwise can be an overwhelming volume of research, confusion, fear, sadness, heartache, loneliness, anger, joy, love, and sheer emotional and physical exhaustion. I can also confirm for you that life goes on, with all its demands, additional responsibilities, and pleasures, despite your individual situation.

Author's note: Occasionally, when quoting sources that are from earlier times, I've included terms or language that today might be antiquated or deemed inappropriate. Please be assured that no offense is intended; this is only to ensure these sources are quoted accurately.

CHAPTER 1

REGRESSION AND CONFUSION

• • • • • • • • • • •

It's spring in the mid-Atlantic. The dogwoods and azaleas have finished blooming, and everything is green after months of cold, dark skies. To my mind, the only positive aspect of winter is a warm fireplace and occasionally a ski slope. In the spring, I can plant my garden, feel the warmth of the sun, and absorb the renewed energy that comes with the season.

Spring brings morning tea on the back porch and a glass of wine in the evening, while taking in the beauty and tranquility of my backyard. Being a more-than-full-time working mother, my porch and garden are a meditative escape. I feel grounded there. It's a place of reflection where I often contemplate the multiple challenges and complexities of the past seventeen years.

As I reflect, I often go back to three days in my life I remember with vivid detail: the day I married William and the days our two children, Jackson and Abby, were born. I was forty-four years old on August 15, 2002, when Bill and I welcomed Abby into our lives. I finally had everything I'd dreamed of: a supportive husband who was a loving and involved father; two healthy and beautiful children; a warm and inviting home, although more cluttered by the minute; and a fulfilling career. Like every working mother, I had no idea how I was going to keep up, but I was content for the moment.

For the first time, in the fall after Abby was born, I put Jackson in a program for two-year-olds. It was close to home and only two mornings a week. I thought it would be good for him to have some playtime with his peers and continue to develop social skills. I also thought it would give him short breaks from his new baby sister, allowing me a small amount of time to focus on her during my maternity leave. The woman running the program had a degree in education and had stayed home with her own children while they were little. She had a minor in art, and the kids did beautifully creative projects with her, the kind that you want to frame and keep forever.

Both children were thriving. Abby was growing faster than I could feed her. Jackson, at twenty-eight months, was speaking in full sentences, could count to ten, recognized the letters in the alphabet, and knew his shapes and colors. He was also strong, athletic, and well coordinated with a soccer ball—at least for a two-year-old. Everyone's development was right on track.

By the end of October 2002, Jackson started to catch colds, which turned into sinus and ear infections. *Of course he would get sick for the first time*, I thought—I had put him in a room full of two-year-olds. As books and pediatricians tell you, it's good for children to build their immune systems. So, I threw my child in with seven other little germ vectors and watched them sneeze and wipe their chubby, virus-ridden hands all over one another. I also wondered whether Jackson's constant congestion was caused by allergies. I had weaned him to soy milk when he was an infant, as he didn't tolerate dairy-based formulas. Given the time of year, when the leaves were molding as they fell off the trees, combined with Jackson's dairy intolerance, allergies became suspect to me.

On several occasions, I talked to our pediatrician about my allergy theory, but he indicated that it would be unusual to test a two-year-old for airborne allergens. We had tried Jackson on cow's milk once again at twelve months, as many children outgrow their sensitivity to dairy. He had no apparent reaction, but I continued to wonder whether milk was contributing to the problem. Or could he be allergic to our two cats?

The sinus and ear infections continued. Jackson took antibiotics virtually nonstop from Halloween 2002, through the end of February 2003. The antibiotics would clear up one infection, but he would soon develop another. He was running fevers as high as 104° off and on, and his right eardrum ruptured twice in that time period.

By December 2002, at thirty months, he was becoming irritable. His sleep pattern was interrupted, causing him to wake several times during the night. He began to have a hard time focusing, he was losing his eye contact, and he started his own form of self-stimulation. Although Jackson was continuing to develop and learn new things every day, I went back and forth between finding the changes in his behavior concerning and thinking he was just a busy two-year-old who didn't feel well. He was too busy to look at anyone and was learning to deal with a new baby in the house.

Just before Christmas, a colleague and neighbor who is a professional photographer did a photo session with both babies. Jackson couldn't sit for very long and spent much of the photo shoot wandering from toy to toy. I remember the photographer saying, "Jackson's the kind of kid you have to follow around with the camera to get a decent shot. Some kids are just busier than others." We did manage to get a few good pictures, but it was a struggle—one new to us.

As the county in which we live doesn't have public preschool, I had to find a private school for Jackson for the fall when he would be three—and the applications had to start at the beginning of the year. In January, I took him in for a playdate at the school that I preferred. I watched him play with the preschool teacher and other children for about an hour. He gravitated to the toy trains and had a good time. Although Jackson didn't make much eye contact with the teacher, I thought the meeting went well. I would wait anxiously until spring to see if there was room for him in the school and if he would be accepted.

By the end of January 2003, Jackson started to stutter. His speech had been so well developed that I assumed his brain was working faster than he could articulate his words. But then one evening, while on yet another course of antibiotics, he broke out in hives. He had taken the antibiotic in the past, with no reaction. Naturally, it was after doctor's office hours—all children's emergencies seem to happen at night or on weekends, don't they? So I took him to a nighttime clinic. Since Jackson had taken almost the full course of the medication, the doctors told me to just discontinue the antibiotic.

Jackson continued to be irritable and consistently seemed not to feel well, even when he wasn't obviously sick. My mind started to run away with me. I had gone back to work in early January. Was it the nanny? Was she ignoring him to take care of Abby—or worse? It was clear he was unhappy about something.

Beyond multiple trips to the pediatrician, which resulted in unremarkable discussions, I spoke to a very dear colleague, who is the father of three and also a grandfather, about the situation. He very quickly said, "It sounds as if he just plain doesn't feel good." We were all stumped. There was nothing wrong that we could see, touch, or feel, and traditional blood and urine tests didn't show any anomaly in biochemistry, electrolytes, or anything else they tested. All indications were that Jackson was healthy.

In February, my brother, Ben, and his family were visiting one afternoon. We were trying to play games with the children, and Jackson was exceptionally irritable and uncooperative. My sister-in-law commented that what she saw wasn't "the Jackson that we've known."

Jackson's changes in behavior were all very subtle; they weren't glaringly obvious when you spent time with him on a frequent basis. He was still developing, learning, and doing new things each day.

I regularly turned to the American Academy of Pediatrics' reference, *Caring for Your Baby and Young Child: Birth to Age 5,* to make sure Jackson's development was on track. The book always reassured me that he was doing everything he was supposed to be doing for his age. But I, as well as my sister-in-law and others who knew him and observed him on a consistent basis, saw something different.

****

Toward the end of that same month, Jackson developed a particularly bad ear infection; this was one of the times when his eardrum ruptured. There he was, back on antibiotics. While still on the medicine, one night he came into my room with a fever of 104°. He was crying. All he could say was "Mommy! Mommy!" as if to say, "Please do something to help me." I'd never seen him so sick—and I felt heartbreakingly helpless watching him fall apart, with no explanation as to the cause.

That night, I gave him Motrin, put him in a tepid bath, and gave him a Popsicle. He cooled off, and I was able to rock him back to sleep. I don't know how many hours I spent in the rocking chair that night, looking at his beautiful little face and wondering what was really making him so sick and miserable. Very little leaves us more vulnerable than having

5

the responsibility of a child, especially one who is regressing before our eyes.

At the end of the course of the medication, he broke out in hives again. As with the first time, he was taking an antibiotic he'd taken before without a problem. It was alleviating the ear infection but apparently also contributing to the hives. I immediately stopped the drug, and again he recovered from the reaction.

The hives had appeared on a Friday afternoon. That Sunday, I was standing in the hallway, watching Jackson come out of his bedroom. He stopped dead in his tracks, stared at the floor, and started picking his fingers. I tried to get his attention, but he wouldn't move. After I repeated his name several times and asked if he was okay, he finally looked up and continued on his way. He seemed fine. The entire episode had lasted about ten seconds, and I assumed he had spaced out from being so sick and having the allergic reaction to the medication just forty-eight hours before.

At the end of that February, we had a particularly significant snowfall and had taken Jackson outside to play. Abby was five months old and happy to stay in her stroller as we walked through the neighborhood. Jackson loved to sled, and he and Bill went down the little hill in our front yard multiple times. After the sledding was over, we gave him a small shovel to help his dad remove snow. Though he seemed to be having a good time, something was clearly irritating him. Suddenly, he walked to the retaining wall at the edge of the driveway and banged his forehead into the brick.

Not realizing how hard the wall would be, Jackson screamed in pain. He'd never exhibited any self-injurious behavior before, and I couldn't imagine why he had done something so potentially harmful to himself. He continued to bang his head now and then over time, but after that one contact with brick, he quickly learned to do it on a couch or chair cushion.

In early March, the director of the small, private program for two-year-olds that Jackson attended called to tell me that she couldn't handle him anymore. Although he was not obviously sick, he wanted to be held most of the time. She was spending so much time with him that she was concerned it was taking her attention away from the other children in the group. Although it was incredibly painful that my child was being asked to leave the playgroup, I understood.

All I could think was, *What is happening to my baby?* I have always had the utmost respect for our pediatric practice, but even they couldn't see anything obvious precipitating the changes in Jackson. Nor could we identify any milestone that Jackson hadn't met within the normal range of development. We agreed that we would put tubes in his ears to alleviate the ear infections and get him away from antibiotics. The surgery was scheduled for the latter part of March.

****

About two weeks later, in mid-March, Bill and I planned two nights away alone—our first since Jackson was born. With Jackson seemingly healthy, my sister Mary and her teenage daughter would come for the weekend and take care of the babies. Mary is a pediatric physical therapist with three children of her own—I trust her completely. We all refer to her as "the quintessential earth mother," and, except for Bill and me, no one was more qualified to take care of our children. We weren't gone twenty-four hours when we got the call that would, in so many ways, change our lives forever.

Mary was calling from a local pediatric emergency room. Jackson had had a myoclonic seizure; his arms came up, his chin came down, and his eyes rolled back in his head. When the seizure was over, he had lain down on the couch and immediately gone to sleep. Again, emergencies always seem to strike in off hours. It was a Saturday, and when Mary called the pediatrician, she was told to take Jackson to the emergency room.

My niece stayed with Abby while Mary went off with Jackson, not knowing how long they would be or how long it would take Bill and me to join her there. We were so stunned by the phone call, I still don't really remember packing up and checking out of the hotel to face a five-hour drive to the emergency room.

About an hour into our trip home, Mary called again. The doctors wanted our permission to do a CAT scan. Jackson would have to be anesthetized so he would hold still. We gave our permission. I hung up and looked at Bill, who was driving, and asked, "Do you realize what the doctors are looking for?" He didn't. "They must suspect a head injury," I said. "Or a brain anomaly, or potentially a tumor." The CAT scan would show any obvious brain trauma.

We sat in silence most of the way home, both of us terrified of what we would learn when we got to the hospital. Had Jackson's irritability been due to a blow to the head, a brain tumor, or seizure activity? I could barely breathe. How could I have gone five hours away from my babies? How could I have left them at all? We haven't gone that far away from the children since.

We were halfway home, on a major interstate, when traffic came to a standstill. For about an hour, our car barely crawled. I thought I would suffocate. As my mind jumped from one potential tragedy to another, I found myself gripped with guilt. I even considered what life would be like without Jackson. I couldn't get to the hospital fast enough. I finally sat back in my seat and focused on my breathing to relax and calm down. I have since learned how to meditate—but at the time, it wasn't a technique I was very good at or comfortable with. I'm not sure even meditation would have helped in the moment. I was terrified to the point that I felt physically ill. I had no idea what we would walk into when we arrived at the hospital.

We got to the hospital about six hours after we had started for home. It was evening. Mary was holding Jackson, who was drunk out of his mind on some narcotic. He looked at us and grinned. "Oh *hiiii*," he slurred, waving to us. The CAT scan had not yet been completed, because he had not been given enough anesthetic to put him to sleep long enough to get the test done. Mary went back to our house, and Bill and I stayed through the CAT scan. The results were perfectly normal.

We waited for the anesthetic to wear off and took Jackson home. He still didn't have a care in the world as we walked in the door. He staggered when I put him down, so I continued to hold him for some time.

The doctors had advised us to get an electroencephalogram (EEG) done as soon as possible to detect any problems with the electrical impulses of Jackson's brain. I was able to get an appointment within two days at a children's medical center in our area. I held Jackson while the technician attached the electrodes to his scalp. The procedure itself is not painful, and Bill and I were asked to wait in another room where we could watch through a one-way window. To this day, I don't know why we weren't allowed to stay in the room.

Jackson didn't want to lie down on the table and hold still. The next forty-five minutes were pure torture for him and for us. To bribe Jackson, the technician took away his pacifier, one of his only comforts. Jackson screamed and cried so hard

I thought he would lose consciousness. It was all Bill and I could do to keep from going into the room, picking him up, and running out with him—but we had to get the results of the test. We watched the process continue; the tech strapped Jackson to a papoose board so that he would lie down and hold still. Our baby was terrified; he finally fell asleep from sheer exhaustion.

As I held him that night—and many others—I could barely get out the words of my favorite lullaby as tears ran down my cheeks. I had wanted to learn some new lullabies before Jackson was born, so I bought a CD called *Til Their Eyes Shine,* a collection sung by female artists. One lullaby became a favorite: I played "Dreamland" by Mary Chapin Carpenter repeatedly, so I would know the words by the time Jackson was born. I sang it to him before his birth and every night for years after.

****

It was several days before we had an appointment with the neurologist to get the results of the EEG. The test showed significant seizure activity, which, we learned, had probably been going on well before we saw a visible seizure. I'd never felt more emotionally and physically sick.

I learned that the staring spell I'd seen in the hallway had been an "absence seizure," also known as a petit mal seizure. Within a matter of weeks, Jackson would go from that one little absence seizure to six to eight flurries of myoclonic seizures (sporadic jerks typically on both sides of the body) a day, each flurry lasting anywhere from three to five minutes.

Once the visible seizures started, Jackson started regressing more rapidly. The changes weren't subtle anymore. They weren't the kind where you could second-guess yourself or wonder if you were seeing something unusual.

He lost his speech; he couldn't even say "Mommy" or "Daddy" anymore. He was losing his fine motor skills and some of his gross motor capabilities. He went from eating with a fork and spoon back to finger feeding. His gait when running was clumsy. He could no longer kick a soccer ball very far or straight, and he tired easily.

Even when Jackson wasn't having an absence seizure, he would sometimes stare off into the distance. He would be playing, eating, doing just about anything, and stop—while seemingly spacing out. I could tell the difference between him being distracted and having a seizure in that I could always get his attention when he was distracted. When someone has a seizure, they are not available to you in any way.

I told the neurologist about these staring spells. His response to me was "Maybe he's just a spacey kid." I looked around the office for his diploma, thinking, *Where the hell did this guy go to medical school?* He was the director of pediatric neurology—and "spacey kid" was the best he could offer?

The neurologist diagnosed Jackson with primary generalized seizures. This meant that the seizure activity was pervasive throughout his brain and not localized in one area. According to the Epilepsy Foundation, "primary generalized seizures begin with a widespread electrical discharge that involves both sides of the brain at once. Partial seizures begin with an electrical discharge in one limited area of the brain. Some are related to head injury, brain infection, stroke, or tumor, but in most cases the cause is unknown."[1]

Apparently, anyone who has ever had more than one seizure gets a diagnosis of epilepsy. This was all new to me—there is no history of epilepsy in our family. The neurologist started Jackson on a seizure medication called Lamictal. I learned that seizure medications need to be titrated—introduced slowly and reduced slowly. It would take several weeks or even months to get him to a therapeutic dose that would control his seizures, if that was even possible. We started him on a very low dose, which we would increase weekly. The doctor asked that we call him and let him know what we were observing with Jackson's condition as we slowly increased the medication.

To better track every increase, the dosage, and what we observed, and so I could clearly communicate information to the neurologist and pediatrician, I created a medication table. The record proved invaluable in providing a history of the medication that Jackson took and the reaction he had to each change in dose.

For example, on March 21, 2003, we started Jackson on 2.5 mg of Lamictal twice a day for about two weeks, with no observed change in behavior. On April 4, we increased his dose to 5 mg twice a day and continued to see no change in behavior or seizure pattern. Two weeks later, on April 18, we increased the dose to 10 mg twice a day and saw a reduction in the number of seizures he was having, as well as less irritability. Below is a small sample of the table.

Date	Medication	Dose a.m.	Dose p.m.	Result
3/21/03–4/3/03	Lamictal vitamin B6	2.5 mg 50 mg	2.5 mg	Absence seizures, 6–7 myoclonic flurries per day lasting 2–6 minutes each. Irritable, easily agitated, interrupted sleep pattern.
4/4/03–4/17/03	Lamictal	5 mg	5 mg	Absence seizures, 6–7 myoclonic flurries per day. Irritable, easily agitated, interrupted sleep pattern.

4/18/03–4/24/03	Lamictal	10 mg	10 mg	No absence seizures, 3 myoclonic flurries per day. Not as irritable or easily agitated, interrupted sleep pattern.
4/25/03–5/1/03	Lamictal	15 mg	15 mg	No absence seizures, 3 myoclonic flurries per day. Not as irritable or easily agitated, interrupted sleep pattern.
5/2/03–5/8/03	Lamictal	20 mg	20 mg	No absence seizures, 3 myoclonic flurries per day. Not as irritable or easily agitated, interrupted sleep pattern.

How did we go from a perfectly healthy child six months ago to a baby with special needs? Bill and I were reeling from so many emotions and so much heartache. It was unfathomable that I would find myself titrating seizure medication and facing research in this medical and educational world, formerly unknown to me. All we knew at this point was that Jackson had suffered from multiple ear and sinus infections, took antibiotics, and now had seizures.

CHAPTER 2

BROKEN

· · · · · · · · · · ·

It wasn't possible for me to work full-time while I tried to find the right doctors to get Jackson's seizures under control. I was also on a consistent search for the appropriate therapy groups and teachers to help us. I couldn't leave a child as sick as Jackson with our nanny, but I was glad I had her to help me with him. She also helped in caring for Abby.

I was fortunate to work for an international organization with generous benefits that included a new family emergency leave policy, issued at just about the time Jackson was at his sickest. I documented our situation, submitted a request to use the new policy, and was granted two months of leave with full pay.

I had also just changed jobs within my place of employment, and I was incredibly lucky to have a new and understanding boss who looked at our relationship as a long-term commitment. I changed jobs only one time, due to a superior who didn't understand how I had to manage my time as a working mother. The responsibility, time commitment, and dedication it takes to raise a typically developing child, much less one with special needs, seemed to be out of that particular person's grasp.

One evening, four days into my two-month leave, Bill had Jackson in the bathtub, and I had just finished feeding Abby. I was carrying all nine little months of her down a short flight of stairs, Abby in my left arm and a bouncy seat in the other. I slipped and fell, threw the seat so I could hold onto Abby, and landed on my back at the bottom of the stairs, with Abby on top of me. To cushion Abby from the fall and avoid dropping her,

I held her firmly and didn't brace myself in any way. She was screaming, and I couldn't move from the pain. I called for Bill, and he came running, with Jackson still dripping. Abby wasn't hurt, but I had fractured my right ankle.

Some say that a physical reaction is typically related to a mental or emotional reaction, and you can't have one without the other. A broken or sprained ankle could mean you don't want to move forward in life, or you don't want to move in a certain direction. Clearly, I didn't want to move in the direction I thought we might be headed. I wanted to turn the clock back six months and surround myself with maternal bliss. Instead, I spent the next six weeks on crutches, attending physical therapy, searching the internet (continuing to scare myself to death), and taking Jackson from doctor to therapist and back to doctor again.

The neurologist had suggested that I contact a service called Child Find and have Jackson evaluated for preschool services in the county. The county where we lived provided educational programs for preschool-age children with special needs but not for those developing typically.

This was the first I'd ever heard of Child Find or such services. I had no idea what it was, how to contact them, or what their programs were about. The doctor handed me a brochure and sent me on my way.

I went home and looked up Child Find, which is a component of the Individuals with Disabilities Education Act (IDEA). Child Find requires all states to identify, locate, and evaluate children with disabilities, from birth to twenty-one.

> The Individuals with Disabilities Education Act (IDEA) is a law that makes available a free appropriate public education to eligible children with disabilities throughout the nation and

ensures special education and related services to those children. Infants and toddlers, birth through age 2, with disabilities and their families receive early intervention services under IDEA Part C. Children and youth ages 3 through 21 receive special education and related services under IDEA Part B.[1]

I called them immediately and found the appropriate contact for our county. I got an appointment to have Jackson evaluated for preschool services, but it would be almost a month away. He would be three in June—and I was hopeful we could get services for him by the fall, for the coming school year.

That same week, the letter came from the local preschool that I had wanted Jackson to attend in the fall. He had been accepted. I knew what I had to do, but it took me several days to muster the emotional strength: I called the director of the preschool program to explain Jackson's illness and to let her know he would need a different model of educational services. She was very gracious and offered as much moral support as she could.

A few days later, the school director called me. She said she had heard of Jackson's illness and that the teacher who had worked with him had "noticed during his playdate that he didn't make much eye contact. Sometimes these things just happen to children in the two- to three-year age range." To this day, I'm not sure why she called to share these comments. She had never laid eyes on Jackson, didn't offer any advice to me, and made no mention of Child Find and their processes, nor of any services the county has in place for families in our situation. She certainly offered nothing profound.

This was a phenomenon I found would occur often—for my family and for other families with special-needs children.

Dr. Darla Clayton wrote an article published in the *Huffington Post* on February 5, 2014. The article was called "The 15 Things Never to Say to a Special Needs Parent," in which she offered several examples of the comments she had experienced. I can add some of my own memories—seemingly well intended but bewildering and indelible nonetheless:

"I didn't know Jackson was one of the children with special needs in the classroom. He doesn't look like he has special needs."

"Wow, you wouldn't know anything was wrong with him."

"Have you had him tested? Does he have a genetic problem? Does it run in your family? Is it your fault?"

"He's going to grow out of it, right?"

"My friend's brother's wife has a sister with a child with autism, so we know what their life is like."

"How did you have the courage to have Abby? Weren't you worried she'd be like Jackson?"

I heard some of these comments multiple times.

In contrast, several colleagues from my office had heard of Jackson's illness and empathically offered their own stories of epilepsy. These were highly educated and professionally successful people who had seizures as children or who had children with seizures. Every one of them approached me with great kindness and a sincere desire to help.

I was hopeful in hearing their stories and the kind of seizures they had, but unfortunately, I found little comfort in them. None described an epileptic syndrome accompanied by the significant regression Jackson was experiencing. They had seemed to remain fully functional on medication, and all had gone on to live seemingly happy, productive lives.

******

The neurologist had ordered an MRI to get a more detailed image of Jackson's brain than the CAT scan had shown. I should have realized the experience would be miserable, as this was the same facility that had handled him poorly through the EEG, the same one who had told me that I might just have a spacey kid.

Because he would be given anesthesia for the MRI, Jackson had to fast. We got to the hospital right on time, but of course we had to wait. Before I could stop him, Jackson found a small piece of stale pretzel in the bottom pocket of his stroller, and he popped it into his mouth. It was about a quarter-inch piece, and the child was hungry. The nurse saw it too. "How could you have let him have that? Now we'll have to cancel the MRI!" she yelled.

Patients under anesthesia need an empty stomach, so if they become nauseated and vomit, they won't aspirate any of the contents into their lungs. However, at this point, I was much more concerned about what bacteria Jackson might have just ingested from the scum in the bottom of his stroller, and to what new antibiotic he might have a reaction as a result. I was much less concerned about him throwing up. Before I could open my mouth to speak, the anesthesiologist arrived, decided there was no harm done, and said the procedure could go on.

The hospital's policy was that one parent could accompany a child into the procedure and stay until the anesthesia took effect. Bill held Jackson until he was asleep, and we were both with him when he woke up. Again, the MRI was normal. In fact, every test that had been performed on Jackson to that point was normal, except for the EEG. I kept reminding myself that I had an amniocentesis performed when I was pregnant with Jackson—and the results were all normal. I knew amnios didn't check for every genetic abnormality, but they could certainly rule out anything obvious.

******

As I tried to educate myself about epilepsy, I found that very few epileptic syndromes really described the symptoms that Jackson was experiencing. At this point, there was no other diagnosis but epilepsy. I found the Mayo Clinic website (www.mayoclinic.com) to be most reliable and understandable in describing epilepsy. I knew Jackson had primary generalized seizures, and I learned that those epileptic syndromes that resulted in regression were particularly devastating.

There were two syndromes that I focused on, because they were the only ones that came close to describing a few of Jackson's symptoms. One, Landau-Kleffner syndrome, seemed like it might account for Jackson's loss of speech. It is described in this way:

> A rare malady in which children would usually develop mild seizures and then gradually lose language, first the understanding of language and later speech production ... The natural history of this condition was grim. Many of these children did not recover speech for years. Many of them became mildly to moderately mentally retarded ... No successful treatment has been adequately documented or consistently recommended.[2]

The other, Lennox-Gastaut syndrome, is known as one of the most malignant forms of epilepsy:

> The syndrome usually begins between the ages of two and six, often in children who previously had infantile spasms ... Children with these multiple, difficult-to-control seizures often are given several simultaneous medications with consequent drug

toxicity. The handicapping nature of the seizures, plus the drug toxicity and the continuous electrical abnormalities on the EEG, often reinforce the intrinsic brain dysfunction and produce a severely handicapped child.[3]

The only comfort I found in this description was that Jackson had not had infantile spasms.

I had now equipped myself with enough information to make me sick to my stomach most of the time. Clearly, I could understand enough to terrify myself but not enough to be able to better rationalize what I was reading and comfort myself. It didn't stop me. I spent almost half a day every day looking for any clue to Jackson's symptoms or any article, book, or internet research that would give me a glimmer of hope in our otherwise grim situation.

The internet had become my best friend and my worst enemy. I have since learned that it's productive for your own education to at least understand basic information related to your, or your child's, symptoms, so you can ask relevant and informed questions of the doctors. However, to avoid taking yourself down a potentially frightening rabbit hole, it's wise to talk to your medical teams about relevant research or resources that might be reliable and helpful to you.

****

Finally, at the end of May, we attended a Child Find screening clinic for Jackson's first speech evaluation. When asked to point to an airplane, he sat and stared at the evaluator. She asked him again: "Point to the airplane." He did nothing.

In the past, he had been able to point to anything on his own or when asked. I knew he could identify an airplane, so I asked him to "show us" the airplane. Again, no response. Suddenly, his arms came up, his head came down, and his eyes rolled back in his head. I was familiar with what was happening—although I would never get used to seeing it. Jackson was having a seizure in the middle of his evaluation.

The evaluator was very kind and sat with me until it was over. I'm not sure she'd ever seen anyone have a seizure before, and she seemed a bit shaken. As for Jackson, he promptly fell asleep, and we never made it to the next evaluation station. It was a frustrating day in that we were nowhere near managing Jackson's seizures, and the evaluators weren't fully able to assess Jackson's ability. He rallied about the time we wrapped up our conversation with the educational assessment team about possible needs and placement.

Jackson was recommended for further testing, including a full developmental and physical disabilities evaluation. The evaluation took place just a few weeks later, in early June, with an educational diagnostician, speech pathologist, and occupational therapist. They documented the following:

> Jackson presented as a friendly, engaging three-year-old boy who was developing quite normally prior to being diagnosed with a seizure disorder. He appears to have lost many skills due to uncontrolled seizures. Based on today's assessments, his skills remain significantly delayed overall. In general, his skills appear to scatter between the sixteen- to twenty-month age level, except for specific strengths in visual tasks such as shape matching, sorting, and form-board completion.

The evaluation was only a few days after his third birthday. Child Find referred us to "the central Individual Education Plan (IEP) team for determination of eligibility and consideration of intensive preschool services that would meet his overall needs." So now we'd been through two evaluations, and we still didn't have a plan or know if we would receive services in the fall. I was struggling to remain patient, not a strong suit of mine, but we would have to wait longer as we moved slowly through this process.

****

My family was being as supportive as they could. All were well intentioned, and some took Jackson's condition better than others. Two family members simply refused to believe there was anything "wrong" with Jackson, one repeatedly telling me that there was nothing wrong with him, and he would be just fine. One afternoon, my sister Mary was having a conversation with my mother, who suggested that Jackson wasn't having seizures but that he probably had an itch in his inner ear that was making him twitch.

My mother had five children of her own who were all seemingly healthy. She had seven other grandchildren who were also developing typically (whatever typical means). She generally faced adversity quite rationally and had dedicated her life to children, her own and others, through her degree in elementary education. I wasn't sure exactly why she was responding this way to Jackson's illness, but her denial made our conversations about Jackson increasingly difficult for me.

The Mayo Clinic website provided some insight:

> If you're in denial, you're trying to protect
> yourself by refusing to accept the truth about

something that's happening in your life … in some cases, initial short-term denial can be a good thing, giving you time to adjust to a painful or stressful issue. Refusing to acknowledge that something is wrong is a way of coping with emotional conflict, stress, painful thoughts, threatening information and anxiety. You can be in denial about anything that makes you feel vulnerable or threatens your sense of control, such as an illness.[4]

I desperately needed my mother's support at this point in my life, and reassurance from her that I was doing everything, as a mother, that I could for my child. She made it clear to me several years later that she was amazed and proud of how much I did for Jackson but at the time found it difficult to engage in the reality of the very hard conversations I attempted to have with her.

Jonathan Singer writes this in the *Special Needs Parent Handbook*:

The difficulties that arise from having a child with special needs can be overwhelming, exhausting and all-consuming. It's like caring for a parent with Alzheimer's, except it starts at birth and may never end. It is very hard for anyone who is not in a similar situation to really understand how traumatic, life-changing, stressful and devastating it can be, and the catastrophic impact it can have on a family. It can also be a financial disaster, on top of everything else.[5]

I found close friends and Jackson's care providers to be most supportive and reassuring, maybe because they weren't as emotionally invested in him as some family members. Therapists, medical professionals, and teachers work with children with differences every day; they can see potential in a child that a parent may not be able to see. Given their view, they can offer approaches to therapies and care, resources and research, and the encouragement that a parent may not be able to find elsewhere. They can point you to relevant resources—speech therapy camps, special education advocates, and books—that may take weeks or months to find on your own, if you're able to find them at all.

The neurologist had suggested I order a book on epilepsy, in which he had written a chapter, that he thought would be helpful to me. It was expensive, but I ordered it anyway and eagerly awaited its arrival. I thought the cost would be worth it, if it could give me any insight into how to help Jackson, or at least to find the right questions to ask. When it arrived, I opened it with great anticipation—only to find that it was a medical school textbook, I didn't understand much of it, and the chapter the neurologist had written was of no use to me.

I wanted to haul it into his office, limping on my crutches, and whack him with it. I'm sure it would have had a magnificent impact for both of us, as it weighed about fifty pounds. My proper and law-abiding upbringing prevailed, and I realized that fulfilling my fantasy would probably have landed me in a courtroom.

******

Lamictal, the medication for the seizures, didn't appear to be working on its own. The neurologist now added to Jackson's treatment Depakote and Topamax, two other powerful antiseizure medications, which I tabled and tracked.

My heart was sinking further as I watched Jackson spend most of his time sitting on the couch watching *Blue's Clues* or *Thomas the Tank Engine*. He had lost his curiosity for learning new things and couldn't talk or communicate very well. The neurologist suggested I take Jackson to see a developmental pediatrician in the same facility. As a next step in trying to diagnose Jackson, understand what was happening with him medically, and provide the best care possible, I called her office and made an appointment.

Never having been to a developmental pediatrician before, I didn't really know what to expect. She spent most of the time playing with Jackson, to see what he was able to do cognitively and developmentally. She showed him blocks and matching games, an Etch A Sketch and pictures—but mostly he wandered aimlessly through her office or sat on my lap.

Toward the end of the appointment, she looked at me rather empathically and proceeded to tell me that she would "pray for Jackson." She went on to tell the story of her own child, who had been an honor student in college but had a stroke. The family thought they would lose her, but she now used a wheelchair and was becoming an artist. I can only imagine my look of intense bewilderment. Was this really what a developmental pediatrician had to offer? She wished me the "best of luck" as we headed out the door.

Three days later, much to my surprise, she called me. My heart leapt in hopes that she'd had some revelation and was calling with a pearl of wisdom to offer us in Jackson's diagnosis or recovery. But she wanted to tell me that "she was still praying for us." I think she had really called because she felt helpless in this situation, wanted to offer moral support to another mother, and frankly might have wanted to see if Jackson was still with us. Even though she was at a loss for answers within conventional Western medicine, I did appreciate the empathy of another mother who had also endured the unbearable pain of watching her child struggle.

We were, in fact, on the receiving end of many prayers. During this time, the Episcopal priest who had married Bill and me and baptized both Jackson and Abby was on a sabbatical in Europe. From all his stops, we received beautiful postcards, each containing a more profound message than the last. His prayers were precisely what I expected from a priest and wonderful friend—not what I expected from a developmental pediatrician.

Jackson was still not improving on the three seizure meds he was taking, and the neurologist was becoming less responsive to my phone calls and questions. We were going up and down on doses of multiple medications and changing too many variables at one time for me to be able to tell which medications, or what dose of which medication, were helping and what wasn't helping at all.

At one point, the neurologist had Jackson on such an unusual dose of one medication that I was opening capsules and trying to divide the doses myself. I knew the dose couldn't be accurate, as many of these capsules are not in powder form but have tiny particles in them that are perfectly round and roll all over the surface on which you're trying to divide them. I asked the doctor if the medication could be prescribed in the dosage Jackson needed. I was told it didn't come in that dose, and I should continue to do the best I could. I didn't think I was doing the best I could and realized I could probably do better with a different neurologist.

Most importantly, I thought Jackson could do better with a different neurologist. After three and a half months that felt much longer, I'd had enough of this doctor and the services he provided. I know he meant no offense, but I don't do well with condescension. I'm not sure anyone does, and I needed more support in helping Jackson than I was getting.

****

That afternoon, I called our pediatrician and told him I thought the neurological care we had been getting was subpar. He had carefully treated both of my babies since birth, and I knew that at the time he too was somewhat at a loss regarding Jackson's condition. He's the kind of pediatrician who cares passionately about a child's well-being, and he was doing everything he could to support us in finding the right care for Jackson.

He always answered my questions when I couldn't reach the neurologist, and he sometimes initiated phone calls to me to explain some new and relevant research that had just been released about the medications Jackson was taking. He educated and cautioned me about the potential side effects of the medications. His support was invaluable and something I sincerely appreciated throughout Jackson's regression and recovery.

The pediatrician gave me the name of a new neurologist in a different hospital, about an hour away. I made an appointment, and Bill and I armed ourselves with all the information we thought could possibly help the new doctor. I got a full copy of all Jackson's records from the first neurologist and asked for a copy of the EEG. Bill made a videotape of Jackson having a flurry of seizures, so the new doctor could identify the type of seizures he was having. I also made a copy of the chart I had created with all the medications Jackson was taking, the change in doses, and Jackson's reactions.

There was good news in mid-June: Jackson's seizures became less frequent. He wasn't seizure-free, but we were starting to see fewer visible seizures during the daytime. He continued to have myoclonic jerks as he fell asleep at night, and his sleep pattern continued to be significantly interrupted. Bill and I were averaging about four hours of sleep a night; Jackson wanted to sleep with us, and he tossed and turned all night long. The electrical activity in his brain wouldn't allow him to settle down and sleep peacefully.

As I sat in the pediatric neurology waiting room of the new hospital and took in the condition of all the children waiting to be seen, there seemed to be a wide range of ability among the children. Some seemed to look and behave typically; others were in custom wheelchairs, nonverbal, and not physically able to hold themselves up; and there was a wide range in between. I let my mind wander to what Jackson's development might ultimately be and whether we had found a doctor who could help us.

We were quickly impressed by the new neurologist's demeanor. He walked into the waiting room himself, called Jackson's name, got down on one knee so he could look Jackson in the eye, and said, "Hi, Jackson. I'm Doctor Billy." I don't think the previous neurologist ever even tried to speak to Jackson, much less look him in the eye.

We gave the doctor Jackson's history and all the documentation we had brought with us. He immediately invited two other neurologists into the exam room to watch the videotape Bill had made. I watched the doctors identify the types and number of seizures Jackson was having with each flurry and realized, at that very moment, that I had been calling each flurry a single seizure. Jackson wasn't having six to eight seizures a day; he was having sixty to eighty!

The neurologists reviewed the history of Jackson's medications. They asked me where I got my table. "I made it to help me keep track of multiple changes to multiple variables," I said. Dr. Billy told me, "The charts are one of the most valuable pieces of information, along with the videotape, that you could have provided." I was so thankful that I had persisted in keeping them current. It would have been easy, with everything on our plates, to let them slide.

I asked about the EEG and was told that "it was only ten seconds' worth of the entire test and that, given the brain wave pattern it showed, Landau-Kleffner and Lennox-Gastaut syndromes could not be ruled out." We would need to have the entire EEG reading sent to the new medical facility to get an accurate assessment.

That day, the neurologists also told us that Jackson was having three kinds of seizures—absence, myoclonic, and atonic (a loss of normal muscle tone, which often leads the affected person to fall down or drop the head involuntarily)—and that we hadn't given any of the medications sufficient chance to work before the doses were changed. Jackson was taking too much medication, they said, and they didn't think he was taking the right kind of medication for the kinds of seizures he was having.

You can only imagine my anger and frustration. My blood was boiling. I resisted the urge to call the first neurologist and tell him what I really thought of him. It would have been counterproductive, wasting the little energy I had left. It also wouldn't have done anything to help Jackson. I tried to focus on the positive and how thankful I was to have found a group of healers who potentially could help Jackson and respond to Bill and me on how to deal with his condition.

It was at this point that I realized we had let the relationship with the first neurologist go on for too long. I should have trusted my intuition as soon as I felt uncomfortable with the care Jackson was getting. Parents need to be able to develop a trusting partnership with the practitioners who are treating their children and vice versa. Neither the care provider nor the parent should ever feel alienated, condescended to, or treated in a disrespectful way. It's very difficult to think objectively and set emotions aside when you're in the middle of an acute medical situation with your child, but we need to remember that we always have options. Given our experience, my best advice would be this: when it's not working, move on.

Although Bill and I are fortunate to live in an area with multiple medical resources, we chose to take Jackson to another city, to be seen by the best pediatric neurologist we could find. We're not all fortunate enough to have a wealth of resources available to us. However, even if you're located in a town with very few medical resources, every state has a capital city with additional options. Perhaps there is even another town in which to look until you're satisfied with the quality of care you're getting and the relationship you've developed with your care provider.

****

The new team of neurologists thought it would be best to slowly reduce the amount of medication Jackson was taking and increase the level of one to see if we could better control the seizures and reduce the risk of toxicity.

They also proposed considering the ketogenic diet if medication didn't ultimately manage the seizure activity. As indicated on the Mayo Clinic's website,

> The ketogenic diet prompts the body to produce
> ketones, causing the body to use fat instead

31

of glucose for energy. Mayo Clinic has used the ketogenic diet, primarily for children with epilepsy, since 1921. Exactly how the ketogenic diet works is not known, but the high-fat, low-protein, no-carbohydrate diet mimics some effects of starvation that seem to inhibit seizures. The diet is rigid and carefully controlled and must be supervised by a physician—sometimes in the hospital. Ketogenic diets have been used for children who have epilepsy for many years. The success rate is approximately 50 percent.[6]

The thought of feeding Jackson heavy whipping cream and bacon for breakfast left me cold, but if medication wasn't the answer for us, at least we knew we had another option. At this point, we were prepared to try any practical and potential cure. The neurologist recommended that we read *The Ketogenic Diet, A Treatment for Epilepsy.*

We were given specific instructions on how to wean Jackson off of Depakote and Topamax, while at the same time increase the dose of Lamictal he was taking. I explained that I was trying to divide capsules at home and asked if there was anything that could be done to assure proper dosage.

Without blinking an eye, the doctor picked up the phone, called a formulating pharmacy to ask for the specific dose that I needed in liquid form, asked me what flavor I wanted, and asked for our address so it could be delivered to our house. The medication arrived on our doorstep two days later. This was such a gift after being told previously that the medication didn't come in the dose we needed.

I'd never heard of a formulating pharmacy; why would I have at that point in my life? With a prescription, formulating pharmacies will create a product to meet the specific needs of an individual. The neurologist gave me his cell phone number, told me to call him anytime, and said if he couldn't answer my call immediately, he would get back to me within twenty-four hours. He was taking so much pressure off of me I could have hugged him!

It was close to the end of June, and my two months of leave were up; I had to return to work. Jackson was still having seizures, but there were signs of improvement in that we weren't seeing quite as many visible seizures daily. I had a good team of doctors, and we were on a path to get him off so much medication.

I called the other hospital to request that the full recording of the EEG be sent to the new facility. "We can't do that," they responded.

"You can fly live organs around the world for transplant, but you can't get a CD thirty miles up the road?" I asked. The woman on the other end of the line didn't take kindly to my comment, telling me I could come and pick up the CD and carry it up the road myself.

I took another day off from work (a *vacation* day), went to the hospital, picked up the CD, and had it delivered overnight to the pediatric neurology department. My efforts were in vain, as the two hospitals didn't have compatible software and the CD couldn't be read at the new hospital. I asked that the EEG be repeated in the new clinic, and it was scheduled for later the next month.

The new neurologist sent his clinic notes about a week after our first visit. Seeing his assessment in writing was heart-wrenching.

Clinic Notes
Observations: Jackson is well-developed and well-nourished. His behavior is unusual in that he has an extremely short attention span, wanders around the room somewhat aimlessly, then has some contrasting behavior in which he is fairly perseverative. He also manifests self-injurious behavior, slapping himself on the face and then grinning at his parents. While he has eye contact with his parents and examiner, I am not sure it is age-appropriate.
Evaluation: Jackson presents with a disturbing picture: change in behavior, deterioration in language and memory function, and recent onset of absence and myoclonic seizures which have not been controlled with three medications manipulated in various ways ... a possible explanation for all of this is that Jackson has a pervasive developmental spectrum disorder (PDD) which has a thirty percent risk of seizures accompanying the regressive encephalopathy as well as unusual behaviors. This will need further investigation and discussion in the future. Our focus now is on controlling the mixed seizures, and I am available to help the parents and Jackson in any way they would like.
Concerns/Diagnosis: Mixed intractable seizures, including absence, myoclonic, and complex partial episodes. Regression in language, memory, and behavior. Rule out regressive encephalopathy, i.e., pervasive developmental disorder, Landau-Kleffner, neurodegenerative disorder.

The words "Jackson presents with a disturbing picture" glared at me from the page. I got back on the web. What did "neurodegenerative disorder" mean? What I found was *childhood disintegrative disorder* and a study completed through the Developmental Disabilities Clinic at the Yale Child Study Center: "The condition develops in children who have previously seemed perfectly normal. Typically, language, interest in the social environment, and often toileting and self-care abilities are lost, and there may be a general loss of interest in the environment. The child usually comes to look very 'autistic,' i.e., the clinical presentation (but not the history) is then typical of a child with autism."

As stated by Dr. Fred Volkmar, of the Yale School of Medicine, February 10, 2019:

> A child's early history was within normal limits. By age 2 he was speaking in sentences, and his development appeared to be proceeding appropriately. At age thirty months he was noted to abruptly exhibit a period of marked behavioral regression shortly after the birth of a sibling. He lost previously acquired skills in communication and was no longer toilet trained. He became uninterested in social interaction, and various unusual self-stimulatory behaviors became evident. Comprehensive medical examination failed to reveal any conditions that might account for this development regression. Behaviorally he exhibited features of autism. At the follow-up at age twelve he still was not speaking, apart from an occasional single word, and had been placed in a school for the severely disabled.

This case study described Jackson perfectly; he had even just experienced the birth of a sibling. I convinced myself that this would ultimately be Jackson's diagnosis. Further research on a California chapter website of the Autism Society of America confirmed my idea, as it said basically the same thing.

There is so much conflicting and factually inaccurate information available on the internet, through multiple resources, and I didn't have the educational or professional background to be able to decipher medical fact from fiction. Bill and I were anxious to find the right diagnosis for Jackson. But I was entering dangerous territory by trying to diagnose my own child.

CHAPTER 3

NAVIGATING THE
IEP PROCESS

· · · · · · · · · · ·

At about the same time we started to see the new neurologist, I started researching therapies and early intervention. Due to his loss of speech and development, Jackson clearly needed a private speech pathologist and an occupational therapist, and the sooner the better. These services would be in addition to what he potentially would get in school in the fall, should he even get county services. Again, our pediatrician gave me references for several local therapy groups.

I had Jackson assessed by a wonderful speech pathologist. Unfortunately, she was too busy to take Jackson's case. I was disappointed that she wouldn't be able to work with Jackson herself, as she was well respected and had an engaging way of interacting with him. She told me a new therapist would be joining her practice in a few weeks—would I like to work with her? I somewhat begrudgingly agreed.

When she walked through the door for the first time, it was like the clouds parted, the sun shone, and an angel floated into our lives. Jennifer had a reassuring smile and gentle demeanor, and she was extremely well qualified. She was open to alternative therapies, and, over time, she would become a godsend not only for Jackson but for me as well.

For their first meeting, Jennifer wanted to see Jackson at our house, so she could observe him in his own environment. They worked together in the children's playroom—or rather, mostly Jennifer worked, and Jackson wandered from toy to toy with no apparent focus. My untrained eye told me that she had very little to work with. That first session was difficult for me to watch, and I was in tears by the end.

For me, tears had become a typical response. They had always come easily to me as a beneficial release, but they were starting to flow freely at inappropriate moments, with little or no warning. Thankfully, Jennifer was experienced in dealing with worried and distressed parents, so she was able to remain calm and much more optimistic than I could be at the time. She would continue to see Jackson for the next seven years, and over time, the two of them would develop a mutually respectful and loving bond. You will see, as Jackson's journey continues, that Jennifer participated in many aspects of his recovery and became an invaluable resource for me and, ultimately, a wonderful friend.

It was now late July, and we were no longer seeing any obvious seizures. Jackson was still on all three medications, but we were significantly down on the Depakote and Topamax and slowly going up on the Lamictal. A new EEG had been scheduled, and the thought of another miserable experience left both Bill and me less than enthusiastic about our next visit to the clinic, but it had to be done.

It was a night-and-day difference from our last experience. When we were called into the area where they do the EEGs, Bill was offered a seat next to the bed, and I was told I could lie down with Jackson, as long as I was careful not to disrupt the electrodes once they were attached to his head. The last EEG, I had felt like we had been in a *Twilight Zone* episode as we watched through a window while Jackson screamed uncontrollably. This time, Jackson lay quietly in my arms as the EEG was conducted.

We had arranged the visit so we could have the procedure in the morning, go out to lunch, and see the neurologist in the afternoon. This would give him time to interpret the EEG before we saw him. The new clinic was in a different city, about an hour away, and a trip there was pretty much an all-day event—but oh, so worth it. I continued to be thankful I had a full-time babysitter at home to take care of Abby.

Our afternoon appointment turned out to be reassuring and disturbing at the same time. Jackson's EEG was almost normal. Dr. Billy told us that Jackson didn't have Landau-Kleffner or Lennox-Gastaut; in fact, he didn't even have an epileptic syndrome. The doctors weren't sure what was causing Jackson's seizures. We were going to have to start looking at autism or a pervasive developmental disorder.

Again, the clinic notes arrived about a week later from the neurologist, with a copy to our pediatrician:

Clinic Notes

Observations: Jackson is somewhat tired and a bit lethargic today. He is not wandering around aimlessly like he did; he is not manifesting any self-injurious behavior. He basically sat contentedly on mom's lap during the entire session. His eye contact was much better; he came over near me and also looked at the computer screen for several minutes.

Evaluation: Having a chance to see Jackson a second time has been somewhat reassuring. First, his clinical situation is improving: he has not had a visible seizure now in six weeks; he has become more alert and slightly more verbal. We also did an EEG in our lab which was interpreted as within normal limits of variability for age. This is significantly different than his previous EEG in which he had evidence for spike-waves

---

and polyspikes on a couple of sample pages, certainly some unusual wave forms that were suggestive, but not diagnostic, of Lennox-Gastaut syndrome. Clearly nothing in this week's tracing was in any way similar to that.

Concerns/Diagnosis: Mixed seizures now under good control. Regression in language, memory, and behavior with no clear etiology. At this time, possibilities include pervasive developmental disorder (autism) or other regressive encephalopathy which might be associated with a neurodegenerative process, although that appears unlikely at this time.

I thought back to a doctor's visit just two years ago. Jackson had been sitting on my lap in an exam room waiting for his nine-month checkup. The pediatrician had walked in and immediately said, "Look at those bright eyes!" At the time, they shone with great curiosity and intent. When I had taken Jackson to the doctor's office for who knows what when he was seventeen months old, he had played with the doctor, pointing out all his features—his nose, ears, mouth, and eyes, so much so that finally the pediatrician looked at him and said, "Now you're just showing off." Jackson had developed beautifully up until twenty-nine months.

Over the subsequent four months, how could he have gone from being a bright-eyed child and showing off to being autistic or having a regressive encephalopathy? And what was regressive encephalopathy?

The internet took me to the Centers for Disease Control: "Encephalopathy is a medical term for a disease or disorder of the brain. It usually means a slowing down of brain function. Regression happens when a person loses skills that they used to have, like walking or talking or even being social. Regressive encephalopathy means there is a disease or disorder in the brain that makes a person lose skills they once had."[1]

I couldn't buy it so quickly. I felt like we were still treating symptoms and didn't have a full understanding of the underlying problem that was causing the symptoms. Jackson had been too healthy up until two and a half, and I knew in my heart something had to have happened to make him so sick.

I had thought that children with true Kanner's autism (named after the first psychiatrist to identify autism) are usually born with it and display the most severe symptoms. Their parents recognize symptoms by age three months to six months, when they realize their children won't look at them, don't babble, and don't want to be held. But that wasn't Jackson. He had had perfect eye contact, loved to snuggle as a baby—and still did—had great speech and unending curiosity, and was very social. However, his recent autistic-like behaviors left me with doubt and made it increasingly difficult for me not to lean toward that potential diagnosis, especially as I learned about environmental risk factors that could contribute to autism. According to Autism Speaks:

> It's important to understand that the study of environmental risk factors includes much more than exposure to chemicals. Scientists use the term "environmental" to refer to influences other than changes in a gene's DNA. Autism risk factors, for example, appear to include such influences as parental age at conception, maternal nutrition, infection during pregnancy and prematurity.

> Autism Speaks remains strongly committed to advancing the understanding of both genetic and environmental risk factors for autism. One important area of research concerns how environmental influences interact with genetic susceptibility. Such research is crucial for guiding prevention and improving diagnosis and treatment.[2]

****

During the months of seizures and illness and behavior changes, we had rarely gone out or done anything outside of medical appointments. Jackson had become so irritable and easily fatigued that he mostly cried when we weren't at home. He wasn't able to experience the everyday discoveries from which other three-year-olds learned, and this put him even further behind in his development. I knew I had to get Jackson into a preschool program that could meet his needs. Everything I read and every piece of advice I got indicated that early intervention is key in treating a child with developmental delays or learning differences.

We were about to be introduced to what many parents of special-needs children know well: the IEP, or Individualized Education Program. According to the Center for Parent Information and Resources:

> A federal law called the Individuals with Disabilities Education Act, or IDEA, children with disabilities *are entitled to a* "free appropriate public education" *(often called FAPE)*. This means that schools must provide eligible children who have a disability with specially

designed instruction to meet their unique needs at no cost to the children's parents ... IDEA includes a great deal of information to help states design special education programs *for children with disabilities. IDEA also includes regulations to protect the rights of parents and children.*[3]

We were scheduled to meet with the central IEP team in mid-August to determine the program and services that Jackson would receive in the county public school system for the 2003–2004 school year. I received a letter stating the following:

Representatives from the Departments of Special Education Programs and Services and Interagency Programs; a County Public Schools psychologist; a representative from the County Health Department; and appropriate representatives from the Field Office and your child's current school will be present. The Director of the Division of Placement and Assessment Services or designee will serve as chairperson. Representatives from specific special education programs and related services may be invited to provide information about your child's special education needs.

The letter sounded official, and the titles were impressive. But clearly this was a form letter. Jackson had no current school. I had no idea who these people were, or what some of their titles meant, or what they would be deciding. I could only hope they would decide to provide appropriate and much needed services for my child.

Never having been to one of these meetings, and being emotionally drained and exhausted from all the changes and challenges I had recently encountered, I was thankful when my friend Megan offered to attend with me. Beyond being a friend of twenty-five years, she is an attorney who works as an advocate for families of children with disabilities. In addition, I asked Jennifer to attend the meeting, as she was now familiar with Jackson's speech needs. Bill and I thought it would be beneficial to have professionals with us who were less emotionally involved and could be more objective than we could.

We'd heard so much difficult news over the past five or six months, with terms like "delayed," "brain damaged," "special needs," "potential autism," "pervasive developmental disorder," and "regressive encephalopathy," that it was often hard to stay focused and pay enough attention to process a discussion clearly in the moment. Bill and I would sometimes debate over what we each heard when we got home from various appointments. What we typically concluded was that everything we heard was accurate, but we each heard different things.

I was lucky enough to have a friend to attend this first meeting with me who could lend an objective ear. But many people don't. However, there are special education advocates available who do this for a living; they will become invaluable to you.

As we introduced ourselves around the table, I indicated that Megan was a friend who was there for moral support. There was no need for them to know more than this at that point; it would only have made the meeting contentious from the start if they knew I had brought an attorney to the table, and besides, it was true: she was a friend lending me moral support.

None of the people in the room had ever met Jackson, nor were they familiar with his medical condition. However, they did have the report from the testing that had been done through Child Find earlier in the summer. They determined that Jackson would be placed in a half-day, five days a week, preschool special education program in the county and would receive one hour a week each of speech and occupational therapy. As not all elementary schools in the county had special education programs, Jackson was placed in a school as close to our home as possible but not in the school that served our neighborhood.

We were offered bus service that would pick Jackson up at our driveway and deliver him home at the end of the school day. If Jackson had then been able to communicate clearly, I would have accepted the service, but because he couldn't articulate what might go on in transit, I chose to have our babysitter take him to school and pick him up. Although I've never seen or heard of an incident in our county with children receiving services for special needs, I wasn't going to take any chances when he was out of my sight.

I still wasn't convinced that something hadn't happened to him when I was at work. Maybe his regression could have been prevented had I been home with him and paid closer attention on a day-to-day basis. Had he hit his head, and no one told me? Had he consumed some toxin that was hidden from me? Did the virus I had when I was pregnant with him cause brain damage? If I were a younger mom, would this have not happened to him? I thought I ate well when I was pregnant; could I have eaten better?

I'm convinced that women go through some sort of metamorphosis in the process of giving birth that riddles us with guilt for the rest of our lives. We grade ourselves on the test of motherhood, and no matter how hard we work or how late we stay up studying for the test, very few of us give ourselves an A.

As I read in a 1997 article in Learning Disabilities (LD) online by Bill Healey:

> Being told that your child has a disability can be as traumatizing as learning of a family member's sudden death. Many parents are stunned by such news. Receiving such a message can produce overwhelming emotions of shock, disbelief, anxiety, fear, and despair.
>
> Within that moment, research has shown that some parents cannot distinguish between the unconscious wish for an idealized normal child from an unthinkable, sudden reality of one who is not. For some parents, just trying to comprehend the disparity between their desires for their child and the disability that exists compounds their emotional and intellectual efforts to adjust to the situation. They may feel grief, depression, or shame ... These thoughts represent an all-encompassing need to achieve inner peace.[4]

Every individual and family is dealing with some issue or another; it's part of the human condition. None of us are unscathed. It took many years for me to conclude that Jackson's illness wasn't my fault, and I didn't cause it.

****

After the IEP meeting, I remember being struck by how mechanical the process was and by how little these people seemed to care about my child—at least on the surface and from my perspective. They seemed to lump every child into the same category. It seemed as if the purpose of the meeting was to provide as little as possible for my child while staying within the limits of the law. If Megan hadn't been there to ask the right questions, I'm not sure I would have been promised what Jackson needed.

Megan knew what was required for an IEP in the county, for example: specific and achievable goals had to be established to measure Jackson's progress; he required a specific number of hours with a special educator. What was the teacher-to-student ratio in the preschool classroom? During the time he wasn't with a special educator, would he get support from a para-educator (a teacher's aide for special education)? What would be the range of disabilities in the classroom? Would Jackson have a peer group? How much speech therapy was required of the county for a child whose development was affected by a language-processing problem? How much occupational or physical therapy was required for a child with poor fine and gross motor skills or low muscle tone? What would his goals be for developing social skills or the ability to follow one-, two-, or three-step directions?

Again, I cried the whole way home from the meeting. But Megan assured me that once Jackson was in the classroom, the teachers—even the principal when necessary—would take care of him and provide him with what he needed.

Most teachers sincerely care about the development of our children. They are a very special breed of individual. To this day, I don't know why teacher's salaries aren't on a level with doctors and lawyers. They, too, are required to have advanced degrees (at least in our state), and we trust them with our children's intellectual, emotional, and social growth and development and with their safety every day.

I get up to face two children every morning. I can only imagine what it would be like to walk into a classroom with twenty-five to thirty of them staring me in the face—I'd have to breathe into a paper bag. Most teachers deserve much more respect and appreciation than society gives them today. I recently saw a post on a friend's Facebook page that said, "Teachers make all other professions possible." No truer words were ever spoken.

Megan's assurances to me held true. Jackson's preschool teacher, Miss Rebecca, was fantastic. The creativity and energy the woman possessed was almost superhuman. The classroom had a one-way window from which the children could be observed. I went about once a month to see how Jackson was interacting at school. It was mostly depressing to watch him sit in the teacher's lap for most of the day with a weighted vest around his shoulders, oblivious to what was being taught.

Jackson had developed sensory integration issues, and we found that squeezing him gently at times helped him to self-organize, settle himself, and become more engaged. The weighted vest had this effect and allowed him to be somewhat present in the classroom during circle time. When he had free play, he always gravitated to the *Thomas the Tank Engine* toys at school and at home. *Thomas* was his favorite television show; he had a train table at home, and there was also a train table in his classroom at school, where he liked to build tracks and assemble long lines of trains that he pushed and pulled along the tracks. He seemed to have no other play interest or innate potential to have any other interest.

Jackson's first documented IEP indicated these areas of need: receptive and expressive language; attention to language and speakers; pragmatics; adaptive behavior; and skills related to imitation, expanded play, self-care, cognition, social ability, and fine motor. I looked at this list and wondered if there was anything he didn't need to work on. The only things missing were gross motor skills and physical therapy, which, luckily, he didn't need.

I asked my sister Mary (the pediatric physical therapist) to evaluate him periodically; these evaluations showed that he had some low muscle tone but was still within the normal range for his age. That fall, I continued searching the internet for any information that might explain Jackson's condition, but what I found described it only in part. Even the Autism Society's criteria for autism didn't really describe him with any consistency: "Lack of or delay in spoken language; repetitive use of language and/or motor mannerisms (e.g., hand-flapping, twirling objects); little or no eye contact; lack of interest in peer relationships; lack of spontaneous or make-believe play; and persistent fixation on parts of objects."[5]

Some of these skills he had, but lost—such as the abilities to speak, to display significant eye contact, and to engage in imaginary play, except for his focus on *Thomas the Tank Engine*. He never exhibited repetitive use of the little language he had, nor did he have motor mannerisms, and the other areas of development were inconsistent. Sometimes he loved to play with other children at school or in the neighborhood, and other times he didn't (any play was quiet play at this point, as he didn't have the energy to run, jump, and tumble). He never fixated on parts of objects. His behavior seemed to be related to how he felt on any given day. Most days, he didn't feel up to doing much but watching *Thomas* or *Blue's Clues* on TV.

I tried to get my hands on every book I could find that might shed some light on Jackson's situation and read, among many others, *Is this Your Child?*, *The Out of Sync Child*, and the book on childhood epilepsy that the new neurologist had recommended, *Seizures and Epilepsy in Childhood.* These books were wonderful resources for explaining symptoms of sensory integration dysfunction, unrecognized allergies in children, and the effects seizures and epilepsy have on children.

I also read *The Yeast Connection Handbook,* which Megan had recommended. She had learned through her own research and work that an overgrowth of yeast can make you feel sick.

Each book helped me better understand what might be happening with Jackson, but none completely described his symptoms. I was beginning to realize that we were probably facing multiple variables in diagnosis and potential recovery, if recovery were even possible. I didn't want a diagnosis of a condition that might be permanent; I wanted something that could be treated. I wanted my healthy baby back as quickly as possible.

CHAPTER 4

LEAKY GUT

· · · · · · · · · · · ·

I'd been back at work for about a month and a half, having lunch with my friend Sarah, when the discussion turned to Jackson and how he was doing. It seemed that all my discussions turned to Jackson, always in hope that someone could offer insight into what might be causing his illness or lead to another resource that might be able to help us. This time, my hope was answered. I will always be grateful to Sarah for recommending Suzie, a special education advocate and consultant she had worked with in supporting her own child.

I needed someone to help me who knew age-appropriate developmental milestones and could make sure I had Jackson in every program he needed for early intervention. And I didn't want to navigate another IEP meeting without a professional who knew the county curriculum and the school system, as well as what was required of each by law. I contacted Suzie, and we agreed to set up an appointment for her to observe Jackson in his classroom setting.

By December, Jackson had been in school for three months—and seizure-free for five. He was starting to talk a little more, regaining some of his words, and stringing two- to four-word sentences together. But he still didn't ever seem to have a good day. He wasn't the happy baby he had been; he wasn't inquisitive about or interested in most things; he tired easily and became irritable if he didn't have a lot of downtime.

I sat behind the one-way window at school and watched as Suzie observed and played trains with Jackson for about an hour and a half. When she was done, she came out of the classroom to talk to me.

While playing with Jackson, Suzie had observed his ears turn bright red several times and then return to his normal flesh color. Her first question was, "Is Jackson an allergic kid?"

I told her he was—and that I had wondered all along if allergies were playing a part in Jackson's regression. The second thing she said to me was: "I've seen other children like Jackson."

Then she asked, "Did Jackson take significant amounts of antibiotics before he got sick?"

Of course. I told her about his ear and sinus infections and his allergic reactions to antibiotics. "Allergies probably contributed to the ear and sinus infections to begin with," I suggested.

Then came the profound moment that Bill and I had been waiting for.

"I'm not a doctor," Suzie cautioned. "But I think Jackson could have a leaky gut. Do you know what that is?"

"No, I've never heard of it," I said.

Suzie explained that some research has shown that "the intestines can become damaged by antibiotics, as they are not selective in the bacteria they kill. They can damage the symbiotic relationship of bacteria and microbes in the intestine, causing gut dysbiosis (an imbalance of bacteria and fungi in the intestine). The chemicals produced by excessive overgrowth of microbes in the intestine, especially yeast, can leave the intestinal wall porous, allowing toxins to get into the bloodstream." The condition can also be known as permeable intestine.

My mind raced. "Have you ever seen a child recover from this condition?"

It was possible, she said. "But it could take a long time."

My mind was reeling. Was Jackson toxic? Did Jackson have a problem with his intestines? Was this what had made him so sick for the past year and caused his seizures? Suzie went on to tell me that she knew a developmental pediatrician in the area who was currently treating other children for leaky gut and who also treated children with autism. Her name was Dr. Roberts, and although she had a backlog of patients, Suzie was confident that this pediatrician could help us. She offered to call Dr. Roberts's office on our behalf that afternoon.

I called her office later in the day in hopes that Dr. Roberts had something more tangible to offer than prayer. I had priests in that field helping me with that. What we needed was a qualified medical professional. The office was already expecting our call. We were fortunate to get an appointment the next week. Bill and I were asked to come alone for the first of three visits, so we could give Dr. Roberts Jackson's complete history, from conception through the present. She also took a family history, to look for any autism, epilepsy, genetic abnormality, or intestinal issues on either side of our families.

****

The week before Christmas, we took Jackson to see Dr. Roberts. She sat on the floor and played with him for about two hours, as Bill and I watched from a seat in the room. They played with trains, race cars, blocks, and matching games. Dr. Roberts had a children's kitchen in the room, and they play-cooked together as well. When they were done playing, she looked at Bill and me and said, "He's not autistic or PDD either."

My mouth dropped open. "How could you tell so quickly?"

She gave several reasons. And among them—though this wasn't the basis for her conclusion—was a reason that seemed to stick with me. "Even though his eye contact was poor," she said, "when he looks at you, he's with you 100 percent." This along with multiple other strengths led her to believe he did not have autism.

Okay, I thought. He doesn't have an epileptic syndrome. He had been showing signs of very slow recovery after we had his seizures under control, which told me that he didn't have a degenerative neurological disorder. He is not autistic. So, what *is* going on with this child?

In very simple terms that Bill and I could understand, Dr. Roberts explained leaky gut syndrome or permeable intestine.

She explained: The intestine is about as thick as the eyelid and remains healthy due to the balanced relationship of bacteria and fungi that live in the digestive tract. When the gut flora is damaged, that symbiotic relationship is destroyed, and some bacteria are killed off, some overgrow, and fungus grows—usually in the form of yeast. This imbalance damages the intestinal wall to the point where it can no longer absorb nutrients appropriately and can become porous, or *leaky*. Generally, children with leaky gut become biochemically imbalanced, affecting their ability to grow, learn, and develop typically.

Bill and I were elated as we wrapped up our second visit with Dr. Roberts. After months of worry and a lack of answers, we finally had a new path to follow that might lead to the true pathology behind Jackson's illness. What that meant to me was that we might find something tangible to treat.

You would think Bill and I would have been ecstatic over hearing Dr. Roberts say that Jackson wasn't PDD or potentially somewhere on the autism spectrum. But because he still exhibited behavior associated with autism, we couldn't dismiss that potential diagnosis so quickly in our minds. We didn't really believe it, but we couldn't easily dismiss it either. We would have to wait for Dr. Roberts's assessment, along with further medical testing and results.

Dr. Roberts documented her Developmental Pediatric Evaluation and reviewed it with us in her office a week after our second visit. It included the reason for Jackson's referral to her; his past medical, developmental, behavioral, and educational history; a family and social history; documentation around the physical exam she performed, including a general and neurological exam; her observations from her play and interaction with Jackson; and the following diagnostic impressions:

Clinic Notes
1. **Developmental regression with seizure disorder (well controlled), language delay, and motor planning problems.** Medical work-up for the cause of his regression has been unrevealing to date. Neuroimaging was normal. Landau-Kleffner Syndrome, a seizure disorder that can result in language loss, was appropriately considered but was ruled out. Hearing and vision testing were also normal. Metabolic testing (plasma amino acids and urine organic acids) were also normal. However, if metabolic testing was done during a time when he was not physically ill or metabolically stressed, the tests may not have detected a mild or partial defect. Additional recommended medical work-up includes testing for thyroid dysfunction and celiac disease. Recent reports suggest that celiac disease has a much broader spectrum of presentation, including behavioral, developmental or neurologic symptoms even

in the absence of GI symptoms. Celiac disease results in both malabsorption and altered intestinal permeability. It is possible that Jackson developed active celiac disease, with subsequent development of intestinal pathology and secondary consequences on behavior and development, including neurologic sequelae (after effects of the disease).

2. **Jackson does not have sufficient symptoms to meet criteria for a Pervasive Developmental Disorder.** The age of onset of his regression was later than that commonly seen with autism. However, due to the presence of some autism-like symptoms, an investigation of physiologic factors that are often seen in autism spectrum disorders may be worthwhile as it may lead to helpful therapeutic interventions.

3. **Consideration of other "less conventional" contributing factors to Jackson's developmental regression and current developmental delays should be considered.** A functional medicine approach investigates underlying factors that support optimal brain functioning as well as factors that may be interfering. Factors that the brain requires for optimal functioning include a steady supply of glucose; adequate essential fatty acids; and adequate nutrients (such as zinc and vitamin A). Factors that may interfere with optimal brain functioning include false neurotransmitters generated from foods (as in food "sensitivities") and adverse central nervous system effects from histamine.

4. **Altered intestinal permeability (so called "leaky gut syndrome") appears to be a factor in the development of symptoms of autism spectrum disorders; it may be a factor in other developmental disorders as well.** If the normal barrier function of the intestinal tract is altered,

substances which would not normally pass through this barrier may enter the bloodstream, with resulting adverse effects on the immune system and the central nervous system. Intestinal permeability may be altered by a number of factors including celiac disease, poor digestion of food, recurrent antibiotic use, overgrowth of yeast in the intestine, and essential fatty acid deficiency. For example, recurrent antibiotic use can result in an alteration of the normal bowel flora, decreasing the number of beneficial bacteria and allowing the overgrowth of yeast. In the setting of altered intestinal permeability, yeast byproducts may then enter the bloodstream. In addition, if proteins are poorly digested and therefore incompletely broken down, these peptide fragments can also pass through a "leaky gut" with negative effects on brain functioning. It is theorized that in children with autism, these proteins can result in an opiate-like effect in the brain. The most common offending proteins are casein (milk) and gluten (wheat). It is speculated that children often crave these food groups due to their ability to create this opiate-like effect. Jackson particularly likes dairy products.

Jackson has a history of recurrent antibiotic use for otitis media (ear infections). This may have altered his intestinal flora, with the adverse consequences described above. The onset of his developmental regression followed a prolonged course of multiple antibiotics.

Dr. Roberts's report listed a number of conditions or deficiencies to further evaluate, which included the following:

Clinic Notes
1. **Food sensitivities or intolerances.** Food sensitivities can often result in behavioral and attentional difficulties. These reactions are not "classic" allergies and are mediated by different pathways. These reactions to food can be delayed up to 48-72 hours after ingestion of a food. This often makes it difficult to identify potentially problematic foods by history alone and a diagnostic trial of eliminating particular foods is more helpful. Often the foods a child likes or craves are those which are most problematic. Food sensitivities are often due to altered intestinal permeability. The offending proteins, once in the bloodstream, can have adverse systemic effects on the immune system and central nervous system.
2. **Essential fatty acid (EFA) deficiency.** Studies have found an association between EFA deficiency and a number of behavioral and developmental disorders. Psychiatric literature reports that EFAs can be helpful adjuncts to medication treatment for a number of neuropsychiatric disorders. Essential fatty acids, especially omega-3 fatty acids and DHA in particular, are important for nerve signaling and for the health of cell membranes throughout the body. Risk factors for the developmental of EFA deficiency include: The composition of the American diet: the processing of oils to improve their shelf life, which alters the fatty acid composition; poor absorption of EFAs; and insufficient nutrients for adequate utilization of EFAs. Essential fatty acid deficiency can also contribute to leakiness of the cell membranes of the intestinal wall. It generally takes 6-8 weeks to correct an EFA deficiency.

3. **Vitamin A deficiency.** Research by Dr. Mary Megson has suggested a role for vitamin A deficiency in the development of autistic symptoms; it may play a role in other developmental disorders as well. Vitamin A plays an important role not only in vision but in cell signaling in the areas of the brain responsible for memory and learning. Vitamin A is necessary for appropriate function of the rods in the eye; poor rod function can affect eye contact. Deficiency may also affect skills which have a visual-spatial component and therefore can affect motor planning. It is theorized that some individuals have a deficiency of vitamin A due to the absence of the enzyme in the lining of the gut necessary to split vitamin A and allow it to be absorbed. In the absence of this enzyme, the naturally occurring form of vitamin A (palmitate) cannot be absorbed.

4. **Zinc deficiency.** Zinc deficiency has been reported in autism and Attention Deficit Hyperactivity Disorder (ADHD). Zinc is involved in a number of reactions in the body, including the utilization of amino acids. The most accurate measurement of zinc is red blood cell zinc, as serum zinc is not low until individuals are very zinc deficient.

5. **Hypoglycemia.** Jackson's breakfast primarily consists of carbohydrates. The rise in blood sugar following carbohydrate intake is appropriately followed by a lowering of blood sugar due to insulin. However, individuals may "overcorrect" and lower their blood sugar too far. This can result in symptoms of inattention and irritability even in the absence of the more classic symptoms of sweating and shakiness. One way to moderate the effect of excess carbohydrates is to eat protein along with carbohydrates.

> Protein is digested more slowly than carbohydrates; therefore, any food eaten at the same time as protein will have its digestion also slowed. This results in a stabilizing of blood glucose levels and often results in improvement in behaviors.
>
> 6. **Adverse central nervous system effects from histamine.** Jackson has chronic nasal congestion and sneezing and has an allergic appearance on physical examination. Histamine has both local tissue effects and effects on the central nervous system. Central nervous system effects from histamine can vary widely and may include inattention, irritability, sensory sensitivities, and obsessive-compulsive behaviors. Traditional anti-histamines treat the local tissue effects from the binding of histamine to tissues; however, they do not block the continued production of histamine. There are a number of herbs that treat the local tissue effects and also stabilize the mast cells, thus decreasing the production of histamine. This lowers the circulating blood level of histamine and often results in decreased central nervous system effects.

During that third visit, Dr. Roberts recommended an additional medical workup to include testing for celiac disease or gluten sensitivity, lead level, thyroid function, vitamin A level, and red blood cell zinc. She thought repeat metabolic testing with quantitative plasma amino acids and urine organic acids during Jackson's next acute illness could also be considered. In addition, she recommended urinary peptide testing for casomorphin and gliadorphin, the opiate-like by-products from casein (dairy) and gluten (wheat). She ordered blood, urine (organic acid profile and dysbiosis testing), and stool (microbiology) tests so we would have a clear picture of what was, or was not, in his system.

The blood work could be done by a regular lab, but the urine and stool would need to be sent to specialty labs—which do not accept insurance. We would have to pay out of pocket and bill our insurance company separately. The organic acid test would be completed at Great Plains Lab in Kansas, where Dr. William Shaw had created patented tests that potentially would show the results we were looking for. In compiling current research and information on medical therapies used for the treatment of autism and PDD, Dr. Shaw has published multiple works including "Autism Beyond the Basics: Treating Autism Spectrum Disorders and Biological Treatments for Autism" and "PDD: Causes and Biomedical Therapies for Autism and PDD." His testing goes well beyond examining patients with autism to look at ADHD, allergies, immune deficiencies, and many other health issues.

Dr. Roberts also recommended three books—ones I hadn't yet read: *Unraveling the Mystery of Autism and Pervasive Developmental Disorder*, *Special Diets for Special Kids*, and *Detoxification and Healing*, all of which were helpful to me.

****

This was such a new world for us; I finally had a potential concrete diagnosis to hold on to. As had become my habit, I started researching leaky gut syndrome, only to find very little information from recognized sources (at the time). I did most of my research on the Great Plains Lab website and learned this:

> The number of microorganisms in the GI tract approaches the total number of cells in the body. Approximately 500 species of bacteria are present, of which 30–40 species of bacteria predominate, including several species of yeast

and fungi. The greatest number of species are anaerobic or facultative anaerobes. Yeast/fungi and Clostridia species are widely known to accompany the use of broad-spectrum antibiotics. Furthermore, recent research indicates that the growth of certain Candida types is markedly stimulated by antibiotic addition to the culture media. Books like The Yeast Connection and Yeast Syndrome have spread the knowledge about the health effects of Candida to the general public but are widely ignored by a large segment of the medical community.[1]

Prior to receiving any test results, Dr. Roberts started Jackson on natural antihistamines. We introduced an allergy tonic, which, Dr. Roberts explained, was typically used for colds, flu, congestion, and most allergy conditions, whether airborne or food based. To put it in simple terms, the tonic acted as an expectorant, rehydrating and thinning old mucus in the sinuses and lungs, so it could drain. The old mucus can have microorganisms such as viruses, molds, fungi, and bacteria embedded in it, which can cause repeated infections.

It also reduced the amount of histamine being produced, minimizing associated symptoms such as itchy eyes and skin, runny nose, redness, and stuffiness. But what many don't realize is that a histamine overload can also create behavioral effects: irritability, agitation, restlessness, inattentiveness, and changes in sleep patterns; it can make it hard to get a deep and full night's sleep.

I got the tonic in liquid form from an apothecary and mixed a small amount into Jackson's juice each day. Along with the allergy tonic, Jackson started on quercetin, a bioflavonoid that functions as a natural antihistamine. Bioflavonoids are found in the skin of some red or purple foods, such as apples, blueberries, apricots, raspberries, strawberries, black beans, and red cabbage.

Everything we introduced into Jackson's system, we introduced slowly. After about two weeks on quercetin, it was time to start decreasing casein, a protein found in dairy products. If we changed too many variables at one time, we wouldn't know what was working and what wasn't. So we didn't take him off dairy completely at this point. I started by removing the obvious offenders: cow's milk, butter, yogurt, and cheese. We replaced cow's milk with almond milk. I didn't start reading labels at this point, so he was still getting dairy as an ingredient in other foods.

Because the seizures had affected Jackson's sense of smell and taste, he would no longer eat broccoli or other green leafy vegetables that are great sources of calcium. Without dairy products and alternative sources of calcium, we ultimately put him on a supplement to make sure he got what he needed.

Based on studies that suggest that children who eat a combination of protein and carbohydrates have improved attention and academic performance when compared to those who eat carbohydrates alone, we increased his protein, especially at breakfast. We were waiting for the results of his celiac test before eliminating gluten from Jackson's diet. According to the Great Plains Lab at the time of this writing, some parents choose to eliminate foods even if there isn't a documented allergy:

> Intolerance to certain foods, especially gluten and
> casein, is a common occurrence among children
> with developmental delays. Before adopting an

elimination diet, however, many parents consult an allergist to determine if the diet is necessary. Surprisingly, after extensive scratch testing, the child is often found not to be allergic to any foods. Some parents choose to eliminate gluten and casein proteins anyway, and find their youngster responds with improved attention, sleep and/or language skills. How is this improvement possible if the child was not allergic in the first place? The answer lies in understanding the difference between allergies and other types of chemical reactions within the body.[2]

Another important addition to Jackson's diet was an omega-3 fatty acid supplement. The brain is 60 percent fat, I had learned, and fatty acids make up a large percentage of nerve membranes and the myelin sheath (the fatty insulation that surrounds the core of a nerve fiber that facilitates the transmission of nerve impulses). For nerve signals to be sent effectively, specific fatty acids are needed to bind neurotransmitters with their receptors, which is necessary for nerve signals to be sent. Studies have shown essential fatty acid deficiencies in children with ADHD.

At this point, we hadn't performed all the tests on Jackson that Dr. Roberts had recommended and ordered. Without all testing, we didn't have the big health picture, and we didn't know exactly how to move forward. Removing obvious dairy offenders, treating allergies, and providing Jackson's brain with omega-3 fatty acids were things we would have done regardless of the test results. We hadn't been treating him with Dr. Roberts's recommendations long enough at this point to see any improvement in his health from alleviation of a potential toxin overload.

But with the resolution of the seizures and most seizure activity, Jackson was showing improvement. He was more alert and more active. Through his preschool program, he was relearning some knowledge and skills. Names of colors were coming back to him, for instance; he was speaking a bit more, and his interests were expanding—but not by much. He was still quite sick and significantly delayed, and he had a long way to go to catch up with his peers. Even though the seizures were being managed with medication, we still didn't have a definitive answer on what was causing them or what was making Jackson sick.

****

After we had completed the testing Dr. Roberts had ordered, but before we got the results, we had a follow-up appointment with the neurologist. It was now mid-January and only about two weeks since our third visit with Dr. Roberts. We caught the neurologist up on the approach we were taking and the testing being done. He knew of Dr. Roberts's work with children with autism and other conditions; he had referred patients to her himself, and he was supportive.

Not only did the neurologist work in the pediatric epilepsy clinic of his hospital, he also worked with the hospital's pediatric autism program. Although he affirmed our current course of action, he laid down two rules. The first: do no harm to Jackson in trying alternative therapies. The second: don't destroy your bank account. Some families, he told us, spend hundreds of thousands of dollars to no avail in trying to recover their children. The National Council of State Legislators website states the following:

> There is no cure for autism, but it is a treatable condition. Most health professionals agree

that early intervention treatment programs are important. Treatment options may include behavioral and educational interventions, complementary and alternative medicine, dietary changes or medications to manage or relieve the symptoms of autism.[3]

A Harvard School of Public Health study estimates "it costs $3.2 million to care for an autistic person over a lifetime. Families may spend more than $67,000 a year to cover direct medical and nonmedical expenses, not counting the emotional toll of such a condition."[4]

Add the cost of day care for these children with working parents and, in some cases, private schools, and you're suddenly well past that documented $67,000-per-year mark. What this means is that some children get the full breadth of care that can help them, and others don't. That's yet another reason to recognize that some of these children may not be autistic and to make available the care they need to help them reach their full potential. What is really causing their regression, delays, and illness? What if we're matching the wrong kinds of support to people with very different needs? What are the kinds of support they truly need?

"It is estimated that treatment and care for individuals with ASDs cost $126 billion per year in the U.S."[5] This is a monumental cost for our society and taxpayers to sustain over time. I suspect that as more children are put on the spectrum, these numbers will increase. How long can we afford to do this—and who suffers when we do?

Bill and I were beyond grateful that we were both fully employed with job security (at least as much job security as anyone has). We had good health insurance that covered most medical expenses but not all. For instance, many specialists in private practice will no longer bill insurance companies. Patients have to pay up front and handle reimbursement themselves. I blame this on the overly bureaucratic and poorly regulated insurance industry, not on the medical field.

For us, neurological services were covered, but other types of services weren't. We submitted claims to our insurance company ourselves for developmental pediatric care, speech therapy, and occupational therapy. The paperwork burden was significant—and came on top of needing to get Jackson to private speech therapy and occupational therapy, both twice a week. This added up to four medical claims a week to keep track of and process. Also, claims submitted by a patient are not covered at the same rate as those submitted by a doctor's office or medical institution. The first thing to go by the wayside was most of the monthly savings plan Bill and I had been committed to; we couldn't manage it anymore.

We also needed in-home childcare for Jackson—because what day care would take a child having sixty to eighty seizures a day? We had to keep a nanny at a significant cost, especially after you added health care and taxes to the package. What do families do that don't have these means? I often wondered. As I met more families with medically complex children, I found out the answers, and they were deeply troubling. Some families have to depend on the generosity of extended family members, friends, and neighbors. One parent might have to give up a job or career to stay home, adding an additional financial challenge to the family. What happens with a one-parent family? They become even more dependent on extended family, external help, and the generosity of others. They can't give up the only household income.

****

But for now, we could maintain the required balance of care as we closed in on a diagnosis and the right treatments. The clinic notes arrived reliably from the neurologist, with a copy to our pediatrician.

Clinic Notes
Jackson looks wonderful today. He has gained two pounds in the past seven months and grown one and a quarter inch. He is very focused and interactive with me, showing me his crayons, counting them for me, and telling me the basic colors that he has in his crayon set. He is generally acting like a completely different child than he has on the two previous visits. He makes good eye contact, and his behavior and his demeanor were entirely appropriate for a three-year-old child. Having a chance to see Jackson now for a third time, from a perspective of seven months, has been a very positive experience. His overall situation is markedly improved. He is now seizure-free for over seven months. He is much more verbal, much more alert, and we are reassured that his EEG has drastically improved since he was last seen at a previous medical institution. The parents will continue the anticonvulsant regimen and make no changes. They are going to continue with the preparations that they are getting from Dr. Roberts, and we will participate in reviewing her game plan when she sends it to us. I asked to see Jackson again in six months or sooner as needed.

Although Jackson's seizures were being controlled with medication and he was slowly improving, we still had not confirmed a diagnosis. When we got Jackson's organic acid profile lab interpretation back, it showed "elevated yeast/fungal metabolites," indicating a yeast/fungal overgrowth of the gastrointestinal tract. The results also noted an increase in HPHPA, "a metabolite of tyrosine produced by gastrointestinal bacteria of clostridia species including *C. difficile*." The test report went on to indicate that these compounds may have behavioral and/or neurological effects. Tyrosine is an amino acid produced inside the body from phenylalanine. It's needed to produce the major brain neurotransmitters: dopamine, epinephrine, and norepinephrine.

The lab results also showed low-normal vitamin C (ascorbic acid), indicating Jackson either wasn't getting enough antioxidants, or his body was using them up quickly. Another result was a decreased level of pyroglutamic. Low pyroglutamic is an indicator of decreased glutathione. Glutathione is an antioxidant that also supports the liver's ability to remove toxins, including toxins such as mercury. Glutathione is needed to combat oxidative stress (a process, caused by free radicals, that can trigger cell damage) or chemical exposure. In Jackson's case, it was oxidative stress due to his body trying to remove so many toxins that it couldn't keep up.

The greater meaning for me was the knowledge that Suzie was correct in her instinct to send us to Dr. Roberts, that Dr. Roberts was correct in her diagnosis, and that my intuition as a mother had served me well. I had felt strongly all along that there was an underlying pathology for Jackson's illness.

The microbiology testing was performed through Great Smokies Diagnostic Lab in North Carolina, now Genova Diagnostics. Its website states: "Unlike traditional labs that focus on disease pathology, Genova specializes in comprehensive panels that combine standard and innovative biomarkers to provide a more complete understanding of specific biological systems."[6] Results showed Jackson had sufficient amounts of lactobacilli but that bifidobacteria and E. coli were at "lower than optimal levels." E. coli has been seen in lower amounts in patients with gut dysbiosis and will often rebound when intestinal imbalances are corrected.

Most of us hear *E. coli* and think of horrible media reports on food poisoning. But the fact is we all need some E. coli bacteria in our systems to remain balanced and healthy. And bifidobacteria help in gastrointestinal function, getting vitamins from food, producing natural antibiotic defenses, and even getting rid of substances that can lead to cancer.

Clearly, it took every spare moment I had to study and understand all this. I was a constant visitor to the National Institutes of Health's comprehensive website.[7] The site's material helped explain the function of individual vitamins and minerals and was invaluable in helping me understand some of Jackson's test results.

Finally, the blood work showed that Jackson was deficient in zinc, another powerful nutrient that supports a healthy immune system, and that he was sensitive to gluten, which is found in wheat, rye, barley, and some other grains. Oats do not contain gluten, but they may be processed in facilities that process grains with gluten, which may cause cross contamination. None of the lab work showed any signs of celiac disease or the type of reaction to dairy or wheat that would cause an opiate-like effect.

Seeing these test results, I was dumbfounded. Why hadn't other doctors recommended such comprehensive panels earlier?

We were a year into this journey. It had taken me that long to find Dr. Roberts and get these tests done. Why aren't tests for intestinal health well known and accepted throughout the medical community and offered in all labs? And where they are known, why are they largely ignored? Plenty of yogurt commercials remind us that 80 percent of our immune system resides in our intestines. Why isn't there more reliable and widely recognized research completed and published in this area?

And I was left with the biggest questions: Why do some children react to extended antibiotic usage so negatively while others don't? Do they have an underlying autoimmune deficiency that predisposes them to leaky gut? Some other deficiency?

I had the utmost respect for the doctors we were now working with. Yet even today, I question why the medical community, as a whole, isn't educating more doctors and accepting or performing the research required to better support children like Jackson. Why aren't there thousands more doctors like Dr. Roberts available to us all? As a parent with a very sick and medically complex child, the entire process was far beyond frustrating and painful. It should never have had to take a year to find the breadth of help that Jackson needed. He had lost a year of his development—a full year—a third of his life at the time. And it was not only a long span of time—it happened at a highly significant and critical time for development.

If a small percentage of pediatricians could recognize Jackson's symptoms and treat him appropriately, why couldn't all pediatricians be able to see it? Health issues related to leaky gut and biochemical imbalance should be regularly taught in medical schools. So many children and adults would benefit from the tests conducted on Jackson. Why are we not making them more widely available when they're required? My child was suffering, and as a result, so was our family. How many other children and their families may be suffering needlessly too?

With Jackson's test results in hand, I went back and reread The Yeast Connection Handbook to make sure I was clear on all the effects yeast can have on the body. As I continued my reading, I found that yeast overgrowth may be a contributing factor to neurological and behavioral symptoms, and a course of an antifungal like Nystatin or Diflucan could reduce these symptoms in some children. Unfortunately, when the child is taken off the antifungal, the symptoms can recur. Dr. Roberts carefully explained to me that most related research shows that almost all children with autism have a leaky gut, but not all children with leaky gut syndrome have autism.

CHAPTER 5

CAUTIOUS OPTIMISM

· · · · · · · · · · · ·

Under Dr. Roberts's care, we started to treat the yeast overgrowth and restore a good balance of beneficial bacteria in Jackson's intestine. I couldn't wait to put him on Nystatin (an antifungal medication) and watch him recover before my eyes. I was told in very patient and gentle terms that we would have to go slowly. When yeast organisms die, the toxins inside the cell are released. If toxins are generated at a more rapid rate than the individual can eliminate them, side effects can occur, known as a die-off effect, which would make Jackson even sicker. From his test results, we knew that his body was already overusing antioxidants to clear his system of toxins; his supply was depleted. We needed to go slowly and not compromise his ability to continue to learn and redevelop.

We started him on an herbal antifungal and increased the dose every three days. We watched for signs of die-off: increased irritability, inability to pay attention (worse than usual), and general fatigue. When these occurred, we would either back off or keep him at the current dose until he recovered. That usually took about three days to a week. Then we could move forward again.

This careful process called for a new medication table. This was the only way I could make sure that I wasn't the only one who knew what his medications and supplements were. Also, it ensured that if I wasn't home at medication time, or if anything happened to me, Jackson's medications would be given to him properly by Bill, the nanny, or anyone else who might care for him. The last was unlikely, because I never left him with anyone else.

I also wanted the table so we could share information among the pediatrician, developmental pediatrician, and neurologist. It was important to me to keep all three physicians informed and to make sure they agreed with the course of treatment each was taking. The three had such different specialties that they generally respected one another for their expertise and would base their judgment on the results we saw in Jackson's progress. They all knew of one another but had never met. Jackson needed all three of them, and so did Bill and I.

Over the full course of Jackson's recovery, we had two doctors who wouldn't collaborate with the others; one was our first neurologist, and the other was an allergist. We replaced both. Jackson's illness and recovery required multiple areas of medical expertise, and I had to have a team of experts who would work collaboratively.

In addition to treating the yeast/candida overgrowth, we needed to address the elevated level of clostridia bacteria. In March, two months after starting Jackson on antifungals, Dr. Roberts prescribed probiotics. These capsules of lactobacillus and bifidobacteria would start to recolonize the bacteria that were supposed to be in his intestine. This in turn would control the overgrowth of clostridia.

We had to go slowly; again, we didn't want additional by-products from die-off entering his bloodstream and making him sick to the point that he couldn't continue developing. He was also given a supplement helpful in directly healing the intestinal lining, one that would bind toxins, so they could be expelled instead of absorbed. It took about two months to work our way up to his ultimate dose of probiotics. We had to stop and wait two or three times to let the die-off effect subside before we could continue moving forward.

I was terrified that if we introduced more toxins into his system, he would start having seizures again. The theory at this point was that toxins may have been a contributing factor to his seizures. Jackson's system may have become so overwhelmed in trying to clear waste that it couldn't keep up, and as a result, toxins had permeated the blood/brain barrier.

Because the by-products of clostridia are made up of tyrosine, which is also a component of the neurotransmitters in our brains, these by-products can potentially function as fake neurotransmitters that can short-circuit the brain. The brain may send a message that gets routed through a fake neurotransmitter, and it can't be processed correctly, as indicated on the Great Plains Lab website:

> Products of gastrointestinal microorganisms that have been largely ignored in the past appear to play major roles in human metabolism, development, aging, and disease. Abnormal bacterial products of the amino acid tyrosine are elevated in psychosis, depression, autism, seizures, as well as gastrointestinal disorders like colitis. Treatment of this overgrowth of bacteria that appear to be largely of the clostridia species has resulted in significant clinical improvement or complete remission of symptoms in a number of cases.[1]

We had a great medical team. We were finally making progress in recovering Jackson. The last thing I wanted to see was him starting to slip backward by moving too quickly due to my impatience. My fears were regarding what harm that scenario could cause him developmentally and what the consequences might be. Might we have to start the recovery process all over again? I had no idea where the energy, finances, and courage would come from for any of us to start over again.

A digestive enzyme to take with every meal was added to Jackson's daily supplements and medications. The combination of nutritional enzymes was designed to enhance digestion by helping Jackson more comprehensively break down proteins and peptides (a short chain of amino acids). I learned that some peptides, if not appropriately broken down, can function in initiating a number of adverse neurological as well as physiological symptoms. Some peptides could cause symptoms such as irritability, potential seizures, and some forms of allergic reaction.

In my research, I came across a simple yet comprehensive graphic that helped me understand the complexity of the series of events that could lead to permeable intestine (or leaky gut), a compromised immune system, and biochemical imbalance. The graphic was related to an article on breaking the cycle of ADHD on the Great Plains website and shows the cycle in which some children, like Jackson, get caught.

Breaking the Cycle[2]

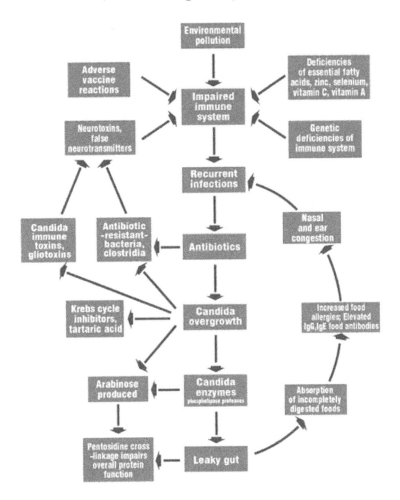

One afternoon, during a hallway conversation with a work colleague from Poland, the discussion turned to our children. I briefly explained Jackson's situation. She said, "I was surprised when the first time my five-year-old needed an antibiotic in the United States, she wasn't given a probiotic along with it." Apparently, in Poland, probiotics are routinely given with antibiotics to avoid gut dysbiosis. Perhaps if I had given Jackson a probiotic each time he took an antibiotic, I might have avoided his illness and regression altogether. I'll never know. But I do wonder why, since probiotics are given routinely in some other countries (according to my colleague), they aren't prescribed routinely in the United States.

One part of this diagram stood out to me: the box on adverse vaccine reactions. Jackson had never had a reaction to a vaccine that I could tell, and he had not had a vaccination in almost six months when he started to regress. I had never paid much attention to research or negative claims related to vaccines—primarily around the measles, mumps, and rubella (MMR) vaccine and the preservative thimerosal, a mercury-containing preservative. As Jackson never had a visible reaction to a vaccine, I didn't think they had affected him, other than preventing the illnesses they were supposed to prevent.

I'm not in any way suggesting that vaccines cause autism; however, we already know that leaky gut leads to a compromised immune system or vice versa and that, as Dr. Natasha Campbell-McBride, MD, says:

> A compromised immune system is not going to react to environmental insults in the normal way! Vaccination is a huge insult to the immune system. The manufacturers of vaccines produce them for children with normal immune systems which will react to these vaccines in a predictable way. However, in our modern society with our modern way of life, we are rapidly moving to a situation where a growing proportion of children do not have a normal immune system and will not produce an expected reaction to the vaccine.[3]

We check Jackson's titers (a measurement of the concentration of antibodies to a particular antigen in a blood sample) regularly to make sure he is still protected from the diseases for which he was vaccinated in his first few years. We also do it to reassure public school system officials that he's not a vector. He has since been given an MMR booster and a meningitis vaccine with no adverse reaction. Before he got the booster, I did research to ensure the vaccine did not contain thimerosal.

****

As I mixed different concoctions for him several times a day, I was starting to feel as if Jackson was becoming a bit of a chemistry experiment. At three years old, he was too young to swallow a capsule, and all medication had to be put into some form he could swallow—such as mixing it into a bite of applesauce. Some supplements were liquid, some powder, and some in capsule form. Some couldn't be taken together, and some couldn't be taken within two hours of Lamictal (the seizure medication); some had to be taken with food, and some without.

I turned my medication table into a matrix showing what he took at breakfast, midmorning, lunch, midafternoon, dinner, and bedtime. I organized the timing of his meds so none were incompatible and included notes in the matrix on what couldn't be taken with which and how each should be administered. I posted the matrix on a kitchen cabinet and trained Bill and the babysitter on how to give Jackson all his meds and supplements. We poked so much applesauce down the child that to this day, he won't touch it.

Below is a sample of the type of matrix I developed.

Medication	Wake-up	Breakfast	Lunch
Lamictal		35 mg (one 25-mg tablet and two 5-mg tablets): crush and put in a bite of applesauce or between two slices of banana. (**Do not put on anything hot.**)	
Quercetin	100 mg. Open one capsule and put in cup of juice (half orange juice / half water)		
Permavite			

Medication	Afternoon Snack	Dinner	Before Bed
Lamictal		35 mg (one 25-mg tablet and two 5-mg tablets): crush and put in a bite of applesauce or between two slices of banana. (**Do not put on anything hot.**)	
Quercetin			100 mg. Open one capsule and put in cup of juice (half apple juice / half water)
Permavite	½ tsp. put in a bite of applesauce or between two slices of banana. (**Never give within one hour of any other medication except quercetin.**)		

Throughout the year, the number of ear infections Jackson had decreased. But he had one or two that made him particularly sick. We saw a temporary regression with each bacterial infection. To add to the concern, we were running out of options for antibiotics, given the allergic reactions he'd had. Although we tried to limit antibiotics at this point, they were still necessary on occasion.

We took Jackson to an allergist to test him for reactions to different antibiotics, among other potential offenders. At the time, we had two cats and wall-to-wall carpet (a great harbor for dust) in some parts of our house. I also wanted him tested for seasonal allergies. The allergist agreed that it was necessary to test him and set up a separate appointment to perform the tests. Bill took him for the tests, and the only thing they did that day was the testing for antibiotics. Jackson showed no signs of being allergic to any of them, even the ones that had caused hives in the past.

When we went back for the remaining tests, I explained more about Jackson's condition and the therapies we were pursuing. Not all physicians agree on similar approaches; the allergist did not feel comfortable with the path we were following and asked that I choose between physicians.

I didn't have to think long. I had finally found a developmental pediatrician who could treat my child like an individual, who could think beyond her textbooks and quickly recognize what was making Jackson sick. She had worked to peel back every layer of this complex biochemical onion and to educate Bill and me—and she could potentially help Jackson recover. Removing Jackson from Dr. Roberts's care, we decided, would happen about the same time hell froze over.

I thought the allergist was narrow-minded, insecure, and intimidated by the practice Dr. Roberts had developed. My sense was that he didn't understand the work she was doing and was therefore not open to it. My impulse was to pick Jackson up and tell the allergist that he was the one who wasn't qualified to treat my child, but I restrained myself. He didn't do the testing that day, and we never returned to his office.

If I had learned anything over the last year and a half, it was to recognize and learn from experiences that weren't ideal. There are plenty of allergists available. We were putting way too much effort into helping Jackson to take up precious time with any situation that wasn't particularly helpful.

****

Not long after, I got a call at work from one of the preschool special education coordinators for the county, telling me she had been observing in Jackson's classroom. Her voice quivered as she told me that Jackson had just led his class in his favorite song. Everyone was amazed and thrilled with his progress. As we started to detoxify him and heal his intestine, his developmental achievements were returning, although very slowly. He was still significantly delayed and, to my observance, very fragile. But we saw progress. We were only two months into treating the biochemical imbalance. To provide perspective at this point, it would take years of treatment.

A few weeks later, I was in Jackson's classroom when another mother, who had an equally complex child, asked me, "What program do you have Jackson in? I want my son in the same program."

"Jackson isn't in an organized program," I replied. "He's being treated for a specific diagnosis by multiple doctors and therapists."

I didn't think she was thinking clearly. She didn't even know what Jackson's issues were, and her son's behavior showed no resemblance to what Jackson had been through.

But as I thought about it, I realized what was behind her question: she was just as desperate for her child to recover as I was for mine. She also wanted a diagnosis for her son that could be treated, and I viewed her with much more empathy and compassion from then on. Jackson had children in his class with Down syndrome, West syndrome, intellectual disabilities, probably autism, and several other undiagnosed issues. Every one of those families wanted their children to be as healthy as possible and have the opportunity to make developmental progress.

By the end of the year, Jackson's recovery continued, painfully slowly. Although he had worked toward the goals established for him during the school year, he hadn't mastered any of the age-appropriate skills identified, and his teachers were concerned that he might regress over the summer if he didn't continue in a preschool setting. At three, almost four, he still wasn't potty trained, couldn't dress himself, wasn't displaying a wide variety of play skills, couldn't attend to a particular activity for a required period of time, was still struggling with communication, and needed to continue to work on foundational fine motor skills. The school system offered us the same services we had received throughout the year during the summer break and for the next school year.

Until Jackson was in the third grade, I never attended an IEP meeting without Suzie—and even then, it was a questionable decision to go without her. Bill and I were grateful for what the school system had to offer. But on Suzie's advice, we put Jackson that summer in a private day camp run by a speech pathologist. He would get speech and occupational therapy every day. He would also have exposure to a different variety of programs and to other children. The camp was a five-week, half-day speech-and-language program with a different theme each week. Jackson would learn about outer space, gardening, construction, pets, and the ocean.

I have to admit, camp was sounding good to me too. I was desperate for a week of arts and crafts, spa treatments, exercise, and mostly sleep. What I would give for sleep! All the research I was doing was on my own time, and I had to keep up at work so Bill and I could afford Jackson's recovery. That meant giving up sleep to understand what the doctors were telling me and to learn enough to ask the right questions.

I had been feeling somewhat robotic as I moved through my days. I was offered a promotion to a higher-level position in a different department at work during this timeframe but chose to decline it. Ultimately, the decision would have a negative long-term effect on my career, but I wasn't thinking long-term at the time. I couldn't take on any more responsibility. I could barely think three weeks in advance. Frankly, if we could have afforded it, I would have abandoned my career—at least for the time being.

Any time I had outside of work was spent with Jackson and Abby, then twenty-one months old. There were no date nights with William or uninterrupted time to be a couple, no time to myself, no regular exercise, and I hadn't lost the twenty-five to thirty pounds I'd gained during my pregnancies. The past year had been lived in survival mode. This was life as we knew it— and I would do it all over again to help either of my children.

I was particularly tired that Memorial Day weekend as I wheeled my shopping cart through the grocery store. There were times I would linger on my way there and home just to get some time to myself. When I walked back into the house, Abby was crying—not just a typical cry but a screaming, painful cry. Bill said, "I couldn't console her after she fell about two feet from the ladder on our backyard slide." I tried but also failed to calm her.

As usual for an emergency, it was a Sunday—and the pediatrician's office was closed. I took her to an after-hours clinic to find that she had fractured her shoulder. We saw an orthopedist the next day, who put her in a soft brace and sent us home. As I sat with her for the next two or three days, I realized how much of her little life I was missing while trying to help Jackson. I started feeling as though I was being cheated out of watching my second and last child's growth and development. I couldn't remember the first time she had rolled over or her first step as I did Jackson's. I know I was there for them, but I didn't remember.

Given that I was forty-two years old when Jackson was born, I had never expected to have another child. When I realized I was pregnant with Abby, my first reaction was not one of overwhelming elation but that "something's going to happen to Jackson." The next day, I saw Abby's heartbeat through an ultrasound. I was six weeks pregnant and was elated by that heartbeat. I put the dark thoughts about Jackson out of my mind and awaited the birth of an amazing new gift—now this toddler sitting in my lap, with a fractured shoulder, wanting nothing more than my undivided attention.

****

The week before Jackson's camp started, we took a vacation at the beach with friends and family. Jackson had just had his fourth birthday, and Abby wasn't quite two. Her shoulder had healed quickly, and I spent a lot of time that week sitting on the beach under an umbrella holding Jackson while I watched Abby play. I thought of our journey to date. It had been a full year since we had started seeing the second neurologist and had gotten Jackson's seizures under control. It had been only about six months since we had started seeing Dr. Roberts and started treatment for leaky gut and biochemical imbalance.

Jackson still tired easily and found it calming, just as I always have, to sit and stare at the ocean. Despite his improvement, Bill and I were painfully aware of how sick he still was. Having a full week off from work to spend with him reminded us of how far he had to go in his recovery. Although his speech was better in that he could access more words, he still didn't articulate his needs or wants very well, and his eye contact had improved but remained poor.

The first day of speech camp did not go at all as I had hoped. A girl who had been in Jackson's preschool class was also attending the camp, and I thought he would be excited to see her. He screamed and cried when I told him goodbye and clung to my legs so tightly I couldn't move. None of the other children seemed to be having an issue transitioning from their mothers to the camp therapists, and Jackson had never exhibited this type of separation anxiety before. He must have felt physically miserable that day but was incapable of telling me.

I sat on the floor with him in my lap for about five minutes and then asked the director of the camp what she wanted me to do. I thought if I could get out of his sight he'd settle down, as most children do, and the therapists would be able to work with him. She suggested that I leave, and I handed Jackson over to her. I could still hear him screaming as I walked down the hall back to my car. As expected, he calmed down after I left and seemed to enjoy his day. He was unhappy separating from me the second day as well, but after that, he went to camp with enthusiasm.

We developed eight goals for Jackson that summer at speech camp:

1. Increase correct use of pronouns (I, my, your, she, he)
2. Increase expressive language skills
3. Answer "wh" questions (what, who, where)
4. Follow two-step directions

5. Increase play skills
6. Initiate interaction with peers
7. Increase attention and participation during group activities
8. Improve potty-training skills

He worked toward these goals over the five-week period, with two speech pathologists, through integrated play, but he was still toxic and mastered very few of them. One positive aspect of all Jackson's therapy was that it prevented him from backsliding that summer; he moved slowly forward.

He continued to confuse pronouns. Some days he appeared distracted and spoke only when prompted by the clinician, and other days he would produce multiple short sentences independently. By the end of camp, he was able to answer what and who questions, which are more concrete, with about 85 percent accuracy, but he was not able to answer when or why questions, which are more abstract. He did consistently follow simple two-step directions but was much less accurate in following three-step directions.

On a few occasions, Jackson was able to sustain play with a peer and a clinician for more than ten minutes but then would continue to play independently with another child for only about two to three minutes. The camp director did note that Jackson was extremely social and wanted very much to interact with his peers, and that he also made tremendous progress with his ability to pay attention and participate during group activities. As I anticipated, Jackson did not meet the goal of potty training at camp. Perhaps there was just too much going on around him, or maybe that's just what I wanted to believe.

I had started to potty train Jackson at two and a half, right before the seizures started, but I had to drop that effort. Children often lose control of their bladders when they have a seizure, and there was no point in taking him out of a diaper when I knew it wasn't physically possible for him to be successful. However, we were past the point of uncontrolled seizures when the camp director offered to help me with it; after all, it was only to her advantage. I had read several articles on how to toilet train a child with developmental delays, but these all seemed rather punitive to me. I finally called my sister Mary and asked her how she had trained her three children.

I followed her advice to the letter. Jackson and I went into the bathroom one Saturday morning with lots of water and apple juice, a stack of books, a baby doll that wets, and two pairs of training pants. I took his diaper off and sat myself on a stool in front of the door, so he couldn't escape. I gave the doll lots of water and held her while she performed in the toilet exactly as planned. We had a party, praised the doll, and I hummed "Stars and Stripes Forever" as we marched around the bathroom.

I then got Jackson to drink water and juice until he had to go. He didn't quite hit his mark to start, but I stood him in front of the toilet, and the party was on. More Souza marches, more whooping and hollering, more water and juice—and the next time, he walked over to the toilet and mastered his task. I put training pants on him and kept up the routine, so he could learn to pull his pants down the next time he had to go. He was successful on his second try, and I let him out of the bathroom. I think we were in there for about two-and-a-half hours. I routinely took him to the bathroom every fifteen minutes for the rest of the day, to ensure his success.

He never had an accident after that. I owe much of Jackson's accomplished potty training to my sister and John Philip Sousa. We'd been working at it at home, in preschool, and at summer camp for a year. I never minded changing his diaper, but he had just turned four, and Miss Rebecca would be very happy come fall. Potty training may seem mundane to many, but given Jackson's history, it was a monumental milestone. At one point, we didn't know if he would ever be able to be potty trained. He was ready, and so were we.

CHAPTER 6

THE NEW NORMAL

· · · · · · · · · · · ·

It was hard to live in the moment and not project what the future might hold. When Jackson was ten, would he still be at a four-year-old level? Dr. Roberts's mantra was: "He's going to continue learning, growing, and developing, until he tells us otherwise."

At four years and two months, Jackson underwent new urine tests. It was just before the 2004–2005 school year, and we wanted a clear picture on how his physical recovery was progressing. The results showed that three organic acid indicators remained high, and he had an elevated level of another one called 5-HIAA, or 5-hydroxyindoleacetic acid. I'd never heard of it, could barely pronounce it, and had no idea what it was or did.

Typically, the lab would send results to Dr. Roberts. She would copy me on them, and then we would discuss them over the phone. She was an excellent translator and very helpful, as I didn't understand much of what I read until she explained it to me. On occasion, the results would go directly to her, with a copy to me from the lab. This was one of those occasions, and I read the laboratory interpretation without the benefit of her explanation. The interpretation said, "elevated 5-hydroxyindoleacetic acid is seen in carcinoid syndrome, as well as in patients on a diet rich in certain foods, including bananas, plums, pineapples, and tomatoes."

I may not have known what 5-HIAA was, but I understood what carcinoid meant. I ran to the computer, pulled up the Mayo Clinic website, and searched:

> Carcinoid syndrome occurs when a rare cancerous tumor called a carcinoid tumor secretes certain chemicals into your bloodstream, causing a variety of signs and symptoms. Carcinoid tumors occur most commonly in the gastrointestinal tract or lungs. Because carcinoid tumors generally grow slowly, you typically wouldn't experience carcinoid syndrome until the tumors are quite advanced. You might discover you have carcinoid cancer through a test for an unrelated disease or condition.[1]

Had the damage to Jackson's intestine and biochemical imbalance now caused cancer, and would he be able to survive it? As a consultant in the health care practice of a Big Four consulting firm—a previous employer—I had visited an oncology ward of a children's hospital and remembered how pale, thin, and sick some of the children were. My heart broke for them and their families. The very painful reality is that children get sick, and some of them do die. I didn't want to go back to the oncology ward—certainly not with my own child.

But for the first time since Jackson got sick, I was able to put a potential diagnosis out of my mind until I could talk to Dr. Roberts and get her interpretation. I don't think this was a mature and impressive display of rational behavior on my part. Rather, the thought of Jackson having cancer was so horrific that I couldn't let my mind even consider that kind of diagnosis. When Jackson's seizures were uncontrolled, I had gone through a phase of being nauseated most of the time, and I didn't want to start that all over again. I'm not very good at compartmentalizing, but for my own self-preservation, something—maybe fear, maybe divine intervention—allowed me to tuck these lab results away until they could be interpreted by someone far more qualified than I.

Because the tests could be processed at a typical lab, they were done through our pediatrician's office. The results had been sent to him, as well as to Dr. Roberts and me. As soon as he read them—and before I spoke with Dr. Roberts—he had called me. I could tell by the tone in his voice that he was concerned about the results as he explained carcinoid tumors to me. This was a serious result, and we needed to address it accordingly. We agreed that I would talk to Dr. Roberts about additional testing.

Although Dr. Roberts also took the test results seriously, she was not alarmed. I had started putting a lot of Jackson's supplements between two slices of banana as an alternative to applesauce. He loved bananas and ate them regularly, as many as two a day some days. She attributed the increased 5-HIAA to bananas, at least in part—and she was correct. Additional testing showed no indication of cancer. We had peeled away another layer of the complex onion.

****

On his first day back to school, Jackson remembered Miss Rebecca and greeted her with a hug. He was happy to be back but faced another challenging year developmentally. The goals set in his IEP meeting at the beginning of the year included most of the goals from the previous year, minus toileting. I wondered how many years we would be working on these aspects: delayed cognitive development and preschool concepts, social and play skills, ability to pay attention, receptive and expressive language processing, speaking with intent, prewriting skills, and fine motor and self-care skills. The IEP also indicated Jackson needed visual cues, repetition of instruction, verbal notices, movement breaks, and brief reinforcement breaks. I continued to rely on the teachers, therapists, and principals who were so helpful and qualified to work with Jackson.

At the end of the first quarter, Jackson's progress report showed a mixed result. He was on track to master the cognitive development goals by the end of the school year. However, there was a good chance some goals related to speech and language, prewriting, and fine motor skills might not be met. Most teachers and therapists working with Jackson at the time had commented to me that Jackson seemed to have what he needed cognitively but that he couldn't consistently access, communicate, or demonstrate the information available to him. If I had toxins, fake neurotransmitters, and seizure medication clogging my brain, I wouldn't be able to think or express myself consistently either, I thought.

One of the teaching strategies with which Jackson was struggling was a new technique in speech to help children identify and talk about objects in a black-and-white picture. The school's speech pathologist was concerned Jackson wasn't doing well in this area. I asked her to send a packet of the pictures home, so I could help him with them. She sent about five to me, each of which looked like a Rorschach test gone bad. All I saw were black blobs on a white piece of paper.

Jackson was four, with learning differences; I was forty-seven with a master's degree, yet I couldn't figure out the blobs. I remembered that I had seen this same speech pathologist punish a child with a time-out because the girl couldn't follow a two- or three-step direction. The child didn't have a disciplinary problem; she had a learning disability. I found the speech pathologist to be rigid, with a one-size-fits-all approach; come hell or high water, she was going to make those children interpret her black blobs correctly. I decided to ignore her concerns. I thanked God we had our private speech pathologist, Jennifer, and let it go.

****

Bill wanted Jackson to start participating in some of the same sports other children were enjoying. That fall, we signed him up to play youth soccer. He seemed to feel much better physically than he had. He was more active and enjoyed playing outside for short periods of time, although he didn't tolerate heat well, and we thought he might enjoy learning the game.

Those who have watched four-year-olds play soccer know there is a lot of standing around, picking flowers from weeds on the field, running in a pack, balls rolling between legs, missed scores, and tears. I think what young children really get out of organized sports at this age are social and gross motor development and not a lot of any particular athletic ability. Bill outfitted Jackson with the required equipment, and off they went for their first soccer experience. I stayed home with Abby to give her some one-on-one time.

Bill came home with a disturbed and forlorn look on his face. Jackson had participated in the activities for about five minutes and then asked to go home. He sat in Bill's lap for the entire hour, crying, while Bill tried to encourage him to get back in the game. On a day-to-day basis, Jackson had been making slow and steady progress, which encouraged all those who worked with him, but if you stepped back and looked at the big picture, the reality was that he was significantly delayed and had medical issues from which he might never recover.

As Bill told me about the soccer practice, I could see this reality hit him, abruptly. He sat at our dining room table with his face in his hands and wept. We both wanted our little boy to be able to run, jump, and play with his friends, but at this point, he didn't have the ability to participate in organized sports, or even to maintain a consistent friendship with a child his own age. The truth was, although Jackson was making slow and steady progress, the gap was widening between him and his typically developing peers. While he was relearning and regaining the development that he'd lost, other children his age were moving well ahead and were on target with their development.

We hoped that perhaps Jackson's initial reaction to soccer was simply because of it being something new. Bill continued to take him to the games each weekend. Jackson continued to react as if soccer were some form of torture. It was all too much for him to process at this point. Bill and I agreed that, at the time, organized sports put too much pressure on Jackson to pay attention and engage.

Soccer never worked out that fall, and we ultimately dropped it. We returned to what had become our routine. Bill and I spent all our home time with the kids while teaching Jackson along with Abby. At this point, in many ways, their development was parallel, especially when it came to language skills.

One night, around the time Abby turned two, I sat rocking her, singing to her, and thinking about the events of the day. I got to the part in "Dreamland" where I sang: "One more kiss, and you'll be gone, on your way to dreamland." Abby sat up in my lap, looked at me very seriously, and said, "I will not be gone!" I explained to her that being gone meant being asleep—and, I agreed, she was not going anywhere.

Bill and I laughed about it, but it was apparent that she was feeling left out. She was cognizant of how much attention Jackson got, not just from Bill and me but from the therapists, with whom Jackson got to "play," while she sat in a waiting room with the babysitter. On a few occasions, they'd let her into the room with them and included her in Jackson's therapy but not frequently enough to make her feel special too. As Kate Strohm says in *Being the Other One*:

> Many siblings of children with special needs grow up feeling isolated; they can lack understanding of what is happening around them; develop fears and worries that isolate them further; feel that their lives are very different from those of peers; and are often given the message that they should feel lucky or special. However, others' reactions can increase a sibling's feeling of difference and isolation.[2]

Abby is a blessing in our lives, and I believe God gave her to us and to Jackson as a gift. As Abby learned and developed typically, Jackson would learn and redevelop right along with her. They played and fought while learning to share. When she talked to him, she insisted on an answer—even when he didn't want to provide one. He had to express his feelings to her when she got in his way. Initially, he had relied on hitting when he couldn't find his words. This gave us an opportunity to work on appropriate behavior.

Jackson's writing and recognition of shapes and colors improved as he helped us teach Abby these concepts, an approach that also helped build his confidence. Abby was Jackson's only friend for several years. For the most part, they had a good time growing and learning together. They'd build with blocks and knock them down, decorate boxes and turn them into forts—all the same activities that most siblings do. Again, Kate Strohm notes how this can work:

> Through their relationships with their brothers and sisters, children learn to express emotions and feelings such as love, loyalty, anger, and rivalry. They gain companionship and support and learn to give and take. Siblings help teach each other with social skills and play a part in each other's identity development.
>
> When one sibling has special needs, some aspects of the relationship can change enormously. Until now, most of the stories we have heard from siblings reflect a positive experience, because those are the easy stories to tell. It seems they are the only stories that society wants to hear.
>
> But ... that is not the reality for many. Not everyone gains inspiration or feels especially blessed by having a brother or sister with special needs. It is often difficult to be honest when our culture tells us constantly that we must be "brave" or "cheerful."[3]

However, our experience showed that if children learn ways of coping positively with major stresses, they can grow from those difficulties. In some ways, Abby was the best therapy Jackson could have had—with the exception of the Whac-A-Mole incident.

When the kids were two and four, they were playing a game, and apparently Jackson had irritated Abby. She chased him across the room with a Whac-A-Mole mallet and smacked him in the head with it. It was a perfect shot, right on the boney part of the back of his head, and it split the skin.

Bill and I were both at work. Bill made it home faster than I could. Off to the emergency room they went. I arrived just after they put two staples in Jackson's head. Bill told me that with each staple, Jackson screamed, "Don't hit me again! Don't hit me again!" We sat there waiting to be interviewed by child protective services, but no one ever questioned our story. They probably thought it was too ridiculous for us to have made up.

Just a few weeks after that trip to the emergency room, I was facilitating an all-day meeting, so I set my cell phone on vibrate and left it in my purse. The school had tried to reach me, Bill had tried to call me, and the babysitter had tried to contact me: Jackson had fallen on the playground during recess at school and was hurt. Everyone thought he was favoring his left shoulder, but in fact he'd broken his collarbone.

I arrived home just about the time he and Bill were getting back from the emergency room, again. The bone had completely snapped in two, but it was aligned and would heal on its own. Once Jackson got past the first forty-eight hours after his fall, he didn't seem to be in too much pain and was excited to see his bones on an x-ray image at follow-up orthopedic appointments.

****

Around this time, we were seeing Dr. Roberts about every three months. By November, it was time to test Jackson again and check our detox progress. The microbial panel showed the same results as in the past—only with much higher levels of yeast and clostridia, along with two new microbes that had not been elevated in the past. One was a fungus, and the other was hippuric acid.

According to the lab notes, hippuric acid is "a conjugate of glycine and benzoic acid formed in the liver … benzoic acid is also derived from byproducts of gastrointestinal bacteria and the chemical solvent toluene. High values are most commonly due to dysbiosis (abnormal microbial overgrowth). Exposure to toluene is mostly due to workplace exposure but may also be due to outgassing of new carpets or recreational abuse of solvents such as glue-sniffing." We had no new carpet in the house, and Jackson certainly wasn't sniffing glue. That left us with abnormal gut flora, in some cases at two and three times the desired level.

I wanted to scream. I'd followed every doctor's direction to the best of my ability. I made sure Jackson never missed a dose of a medication or supplement. If these levels were going up, how could he have been making the progress he was? Once again, Dr. Roberts's calm in the middle of my storm prevailed. Perhaps there was a mistake in the test, she suggested. It made no medical, or even common, sense that Jackson would continue recovering if his medical condition were worsening. We were so thankful to have a physician who consistently remained objective in her analyses and could explain many different test results to me in a way that I could easily understand.

We repeated the test—it was only a urine test, and therefore noninvasive—and it showed that indeed a mistake had been made. In fact, the correct results were so positive that we had grounds for celebration. There was no more clostridia overgrowth; it was well within the normal range. The level of candida was still more than three times higher than it should be, but it was down to half of what it had been initially.

The only interpretation the lab results showed was "elevated yeast/fungal metabolites indicating a yeast/fungal overgrowth of the gastrointestinal tract." It had been almost a year since we'd started treating the biochemical imbalance, and we'd come a long way. We continued treating the yeast with herbal therapies but moved Jackson to a stronger tonic. We also continued the probiotics that had put the clostridia back in check.

We kept an open mind to new therapies. For instance, Dr. Roberts had an acupuncturist in her practice. Would acupressure help Jackson? He was too little to tolerate the needles used in acupuncture and probably wouldn't have sat still long enough for it anyway. Chinese medicine is the world's oldest continually practiced professional medicine; it is used by half of the world as a primary health care system and has become increasingly more popular worldwide. Techniques are built on more than 2,500 years of Chinese medical practice, which includes various forms of herbal treatments, acupuncture, massage, exercise, and diets. We tried it, but Jackson didn't tolerate the pressure long enough for it to be therapeutic, so we gave it up quickly.

Such setbacks in one area were met by progress in others. Jackson's ability to process language had improved so much that he had met every goal Jennifer had set for him. For example, he could follow simple directions with minimal reinforcement four out of five times, point to pictures in a book, demonstrate turn taking during play activity by stating "my turn" or "your turn," and use words to request help and other types of assistance. By mid-December, Jennifer wrote a new set of goals, all of which dealt with improving receptive and expressive language processing and the motor speech delay. She also expanded the previous goals. Jackson would continue seeing Jennifer, twice a week, every week.

It was Christmastime. The year was ending with mixed developmental progress. Jackson and Abby were excited about decorating the tree and opening our Advent calendar every night. Jackson had been too sick the year before to enjoy it.

Missing the wonder of Christmas in your child's eyes is not something you ever want to experience—certainly not year after year. Erma Bombeck once said, "There's nothing sadder in this world than to awake Christmas morning and not be a child." To have a child that is too sick to understand, experience, or participate in the love and warmth of the season that fills your heart and your home can leave a family feeling depleted. But thanks to so many efforts, this year would be different from last.

CHAPTER 7

DEFERRING KINDERGARTEN

· · · · · · · · · · ·

It was only January, but already it was time to start thinking about the next school year and what kind of classroom setting Jackson would need. The only programs that the public school system had to offer were a learning and disabilities kindergarten class (called an L&D program) or a typical kindergarten classroom. Jackson had improved so much that I didn't think he would thrive in an L&D program. He was learning significantly from his typical peers. If he were the strongest child in the classroom, he would not have the opportunity to learn from his peers—and he would fall further behind academically and developmentally.

Our public school system has a wonderful L&D program, but I didn't think it was the right program for Jackson. Though he was five years old, I knew he wasn't ready for a typical kindergarten setting either. He had a summer birthday, and I probably would have held him until he was six to go to kindergarten, even if he hadn't been ill and didn't learn differently.

Why would anyone send a child like Jackson to kindergarten early, given the struggles he had? And where were the programs for children like him who needed some support but no longer needed intensive intervention? Despite the fact that we live in an area with a top-rated school district, options were extremely limited for children like Jackson. I thought he needed a year of pre-K. That would give him another year to develop and another year for us to continue trying to resolve his medical condition.

For those reasons, I didn't want him in any kindergarten program until he was six.

As a child advocate and special education consultant, Suzie was a huge help in identifying local private schools that might be appropriate for Jackson. I researched all of them and visited six, taking more time off from work to do so. Three of the schools recommended to me had remarkable programs for children with severe learning disabilities. Yet they weren't appropriate for Jackson. Another had just started a program for children who learned differently but were on track to be mainstreamed into a typical classroom. This is the exact type of program I was looking for. Two other programs followed a model of mainstreaming two children with developmental delays or learning differences into each typical classroom. This would be an appropriate model for Jackson too. All three types of schools provided special education and speech and occupational therapy.

My fallback was to return to the private school that had originally accepted Jackson before his regression. Abby was now there for preschool, and the teachers had grown to love Jackson's short visits when we picked up Abby. *Why wasn't Jackson at the school too?* they asked. I explained what had happened and what I needed for him in this upcoming transitional year. Although they didn't have speech and OT on-site, they encouraged me to apply again, as the classroom size was small, and the teacher would be able to spend more time with him. The teacher who taught the pre-K class also had a background in special education.

The extraordinary level of effort required in the process for finding the right educational program for a special-needs child was a new experience for me. I applied to four schools and contacted every resource available to me that might help with admission. I didn't have to go through this process with Abby; preschools for typically developing children are abundant. But schools for children with disabilities and learning differences are in great demand. I needed a hybrid program for Jackson, one that would address his need to grow and develop with typical peers while providing the specific support that he needed.

Two of the schools were Episcopal programs, so I asked the rector at our church if he would write a letter on our behalf to the rector of both churches. I drafted what I thought was a compelling letter, for him to edit at will. Another one of the schools, National Child Research Center (NCRC), was my top choice, given its program and reputation. "The school was founded in 1928 to provide a collaborative approach to education in a setting that supports the whole child, creates partnerships with families and is committed to the inclusion of children with special needs," its website stated.

A friend of a friend served on the school board. I spoke with her in hopes that she could help in any way. Actually, I shamelessly pleaded and begged multiple times. Short of a heinous crime, I wasn't above anything to keep Jackson out of kindergarten for another year. Fleetingly, I even considered taking a leave of absence from work and homeschooling him for that year.

Within a month, the applicant evaluation process started. We had interviews and playdates at all four schools. Three of them went extremely well; Jackson was engaged, playful, and interactive at each school. The morning we took him to our top choice, he didn't particularly feel well and seemed flat. Bill and I watched as he never made eye contact with the evaluator, made nonsensical utterances, made no attempt to engage with another child, and played with the same toy for the entire visit. We hadn't seen this type of behavior from Jackson in almost a year. We drove home in silence, until Bill looked at me and exclaimed, "Well, there's always State!"

As upsetting as the situation was, we were both able to laugh at Bill's statement; we had to have some levity to keep our perspective. By that evening, Jackson had a fever of 103. I took him to the pediatrician the next day; he had another ear infection. That explained his behavior at school; he still regressed when he was sick. After Jackson recovered, I wanted to call the school and schedule a new playdate, so they could see the child he had become. But I didn't. I thought they'd think I was making excuses.

****

After the round of interviews was over, I called the directors of each program to see how enrollment looked and how many spaces they actually had available. As I had feared, there was much more demand than there were available spaces. My concern was growing. I was worried that Jackson wouldn't be in the type of program he needed. I was wondering what other parents would do who were in our shoes. Where were the programs for these middle-of-the-road children? Why are such programs so scarce, even today? We shouldn't have to pigeonhole our children into programs that are inappropriate for their development.

The director of the Episcopal preschool Abby was attending was somewhat encouraging about space for Jackson. Although the school wasn't my first choice, I knew Jackson potentially could have a good year there. The other Episcopal school was also fairly confident they would have space for Jackson. The other two schools were noncommittal.

By mid-March, the rejection letters started rolling in. I think the first we received was from Abby's preschool. The letter said "xxxx Episcopal would not benefit from a child like Jackson, and Jackson would not benefit from xxxx Episcopal." The letter was signed by the director of the school, rather than by the head of the preschool. I was furious—not that Jackson had been denied a spot but that any school director would show such a lack of judgment in writing to a parent to tell them that their school wouldn't benefit from their child. What an incredibly thoughtless, offensive, inconsiderate, unprofessional—and frankly, rude—thing to say to anyone.

I called the head of the preschool, who explained that her hands had been tied by the director, and there was nothing she could do. I was so angry when I read the words again that I tore up the letter and threw it in the trash. I wish I had kept it, highlighted the offensive words, and sent a copy back to the rector of that church. I wanted to tell the preschool director that if the school wouldn't benefit from a child like Jackson, they weren't going to benefit from a child like Abby either, and I would take my tuition payments elsewhere. However, it was a good school, and Abby was happy there. She remained for preschool, but we ultimately transitioned her out to public kindergarten.

The next letter came in mid-March, from our first-choice school.

> We enjoyed meeting Jackson. However, our Admission Committee genuinely regrets that a space is not available for Jackson at this time. We received a large number of applications for children with special needs this year. Our commitment to small classes limits our ability to accept all of the children who have applied. We have, however, placed Jackson's name in

our Waiting Pool. We will contact you if an
appropriate space becomes available.

Of course they received a large number of applications for
children with special needs; that's because there aren't enough
appropriate programs for them. I was sadly disappointed, but
at least he had been wait-listed. I didn't give up. I contacted the
friend again to tell her about the letter in hopes that she might
be able to help, and again I begged without shame.

I still hadn't heard from two of the schools, one Episcopal
and one with the new program for children with needs similar
to Jackson's. It wasn't long before I got the third rejection, via
phone one evening. The director of the Episcopal school called
to tell me in person they wouldn't have space for Jackson. She
wanted to tell me herself, so I wouldn't read the news in a
form letter. Although I thought it kind of her, the call was little
consolation, as tears of frustration rolled down my cheeks. She
might just as well have put a big red *rejection* stamp on the
letter of recommendation our priest had sent, returned it to us,
and called it a day.

We were down to one option. I called that director the next
day, to explain our situation and beg some more. She told me
that they hadn't made any decisions yet and probably wouldn't
for another month. I called Suzie to see if she could talk to the
director of the last Episcopal school that had denied Jackson a
place. She did, but the call was unsuccessful. The best we got
was wait-listed. Learning and Disabilities kindergarten seemed
to be looming large.

While I sat and stewed for a month, I attended a preschool
transition meeting with the public school system. They gave us
a handout proclaiming: "Organization is a must! Get yourself
a three-ring binder with pockets and dividers ..." It went

on to suggest nine tabs for the binder for the various forms and background information we needed—IEP, assessment information, school records, copies of dated correspondence, medical reports, report cards, progress reports, work samples, and conferences with staff, teachers, and other professionals.

I looked at the exceptionally large box full of all the papers related to Jackson that was sitting on the floor of our home office. *Are you kidding me?* I thought. When was I going to find time to organize it all in a binder?

The handout went on to offer thirty-nine additional bullet-pointed pearls of wisdom in making the transition from preschool to kindergarten. Some families may have appreciated how thorough the list was. But I'm confident I didn't have to do anything even close to this comprehensive when I transitioned from high school to college. Our papers didn't get organized until several years later, when I sat down to write this book. I knew all the paperwork related to Jackson was in my box. and I could find what I needed if and when I needed it.

The summary of Jackson's preschool year was sent home in early April. I read it, still not knowing where he would be the next year.

> Jackson has made progress across several educational domains during the 2004–2005 school year. Jackson is a different child compared to last school year. Jackson appears to be a lot happier this year and is more animated in the classroom ... Jackson participates in classroom activities with enthusiasm.

> Jackson has demonstrated the knowledge of basic preschool concepts on an expressive and receptive level; and he responds consistently

when a request/demand is placed upon him, which is something he did not do last year ... Jackson verbally initiates greetings with familiar adults and his peers. He is able to identify and use his peers' names throughout the day. Jackson's play skills with his peers have increased dramatically ... When given a choice at center time Jackson no longer chooses the same center daily. He plays with a variety of toys and is friendly with all of the children in the classroom ...

Jackson demonstrates improved attention skills ... Overall, Jackson's attention has greatly expanded, and it is easier to verbally direct him back to the task whenever he does become distracted ... Jackson is very compliant to teacher's requests ... He is a friendly child and is always kind to his peers ... Overall, Jackson's classroom behavior is excellent ... Jackson has mastered the arrival and dismissal routines at school. He independently removes his coat and hangs it up with his backpack ... Jackson is fully potty trained at school. Jackson completes the hand-washing routine on his own, with an occasional reminder to stop playing in the water ... Overall, Jackson's self-help skills have significantly improved this year ...

Jackson has made significant gains in the area of special education. With increased exposure and instruction to complete a variety of new demands and activities, Jackson's availability for instruction continues to improve. He has demonstrated progress toward the goals outlined on his IEP. Based on the classroom data and observations described above, Jackson continues to benefit from a structured classroom environment with a small staff-to-Jackson ratio.

Although this was all positive news, he still hadn't mastered many of the goals in his IEP, and the annual review was scheduled for April 13, 2005. On April 12, I dragged myself home from work to find a letter waiting from NCRC, our preschool of choice. I opened the letter and read, "It is a pleasure to inform you that the Admission Committee has reserved a place for Jackson in the PM Rainbow Class for the school year 2005–2006. Admission decisions were extremely difficult, with far more candidates than we could accept. We are delighted to be able to send you this news."

Not only would we avoid the L&D kindergarten, Jackson would be a Rainbow! Tears of elation, relief, and release spilled from my eyes. To this day, I don't know if my shameless pleading paid off, or if they really did voluntarily find a space for Jackson. I never asked, and it didn't matter at this point. I accepted their offer and wrote a check to confirm his space as quickly as I could. I did, however, thank the friend.

I was able to attend Jackson's annual review meeting the next day with great confidence my child would have an appropriate program for the next school year. During the meeting, additional goals were set for him for the next year. These would include demonstrating increased mathematical skills and attention during classroom activities; expanded social skills with his peers in the classroom; and improved understanding of spoken language, use of language structures, expression of intended meanings, and use of language for a variety of purposes.

At the end of the meeting, it was officially recommended that Jackson be placed in a learning and disabilities kindergarten classroom for the next school year. We agreed with the related services recommended for Jackson but did not agree with his being placed in an L&D kindergarten or in any kindergarten program. We requested that kindergarten be deferred for one year, and, based on experience and the fact that the public school system didn't have an appropriate program for Jackson, Bill and I asked that our perspective be documented in the review.

In addition to the deferral, we asked that Jackson receive county services for special education in our home elementary school, the school Jackson would ultimately attend for kindergarten, should he continue to progress as he had. Although there were many papers to complete, by the end of the summer, we received a letter saying that our request had been approved, and we should contact the school principal to arrange for services for Jackson. This meant that Jackson would attend his private preschool program every afternoon and that on two mornings a week, he would see a special educator in the county school system. We also thought this approach would provide a great transition for Jackson from preschool to kindergarten, as he would already be familiar with the school.

****

We had our six-month follow-up visit with the neurologist in June. I brought Jackson's medication chart so he would be familiar with everything Jackson was taking and so it could be placed in his neurology chart. The doctor took one look at it and said, "This is a full-time job." Actually, it was more than a full-time job. It took three of us to keep up with it—Bill, me, and the babysitter. Other than my making sure we had all the right medications and supplements, we didn't have individual tasks. We had to be interchangeable. We had to know his schedule, medication, therapists, routine, and what he needed when. Whoever was with Jackson at any given time had to be able to provide for him and for Abby too.

The neurologist was thrilled with Jackson's progress and was able to be more encouraging than he had been on any previous visit. I asked him if he had treated other children with symptoms similar to Jackson's and whether there was any research indicating a potential outcome for these children. He told us he had a few cases similar to Jackson's that were being treated through the hospital's autism program, but enough time hadn't passed to document a final outcome.

At the end of that visit, overwhelmed with how far we had come in two years, I asked the neurologist if I could hug him. He obliged me without hesitation. After I read the following clinic notes he sent, I wanted to hug him again.

Clinic Notes

History of Present Illness: I initially evaluated Jackson on 06/24/03 and saw him in follow-up on 7/29/03 and 01/15/04. He initially had a mixed seizure disorder with language, memory, and behavioral regression of uncertain etiology. There was no evidence for Lennox-Gastaut or Landau-Kleffner on his 07/29/03 EEG. I was initially concerned that he might have an undiagnosed neurodegenerative process or an atypical pervasive developmental disorder (his regression was quite late for spectrum disorders), but history has shown that what we recommended and has been done for this youngster has resulted in a tremendous improvement over several years.

Essentially, I slowly tapered and discontinued his Topamax and Depakote and then decreased his Lamictal as well to the current level, and as a result, his seizures have been under control for 24 months ... Dr. Roberts has started him over time on a complicated regime which the parents think has been largely responsible for the resolution of his behavioral and language problems, in association probably with the decreased toxic effects of his anticonvulsants ... Overall parents and all physicians participating in Jackson's care are extremely pleased with how he has done. The only issue that mother sees as referable to possible seizures are occasional myoclonic jerks coming in and out of sleep.

Observations: Jackson looks terrific today ... He shares his interests with me, makes good eye contact, and is happy and bright. Neurological exam shows no abnormalities of cranial nerves. His cerebellar function is normal. His motor exam shows no lateral evasion or locality, somewhat decreased tone ... Sensory exam is grossly intact to tickle and touch.

Evaluation: Obviously the improvements Jackson has made are a great source of satisfaction to his parent and everyone involved in his care. He has been managed ideally and has made developmental progress in context of taking very minimal anticonvulsants and being seizure-free now for 24 months. I will continue to follow Jackson and will not make any changes in his Lamictal at this point in time, and hope to see him in 6 months, doing even better than he is now.

To continue to track Jackson's fungal overgrowth, Dr. Roberts ordered another microbial panel in July 2005. It showed a continued overgrowth of yeast at about the same level detected earlier in the year. I'd been patient for as long as I could. I asked whether we could move to a stronger antifungal, such as Nystatin. She was at the same point and wrote the prescription. Although we were moving slowly, Jackson was experiencing a die-off effect—so we would have to go even more slowly.

The good news was that he was back in speech-language summer camp, and the director couldn't believe the progress he had made over the school year.

Jackson continued to work on some of the same goals in camp as in the past. The final assessment from the previous year indicated that he was initially a little shy and would frequently choose to play alone. However, by the end of the current camp session, he was speaking in sentences up to eight words long and was responding to questions about a story; he sometimes even answered a question for another child. Although Jackson was speaking in correct sentences, he sometimes had difficulty expressing his thoughts clearly and finding the right words.

The camp director indicated that Jackson's pencil grip was somewhat weak due to low muscle tone in his hands, which resulted in light pressure when he was writing. She suggested hand exercises on a regular basis. He would get these in private OT and through the services provided by the county come fall. Jackson really enjoyed playing sports on the playground with his peers and practicing soccer. It was suggested we try soccer again to provide him with opportunities to develop his sports skills and encourage social skills through teamwork and a sense of accomplishment.

After our experience with soccer the previous fall, we'd really have to think about what sport Jackson might enjoy. Bill started playing baseball with him in the backyard. Jackson frequently ran the bases backward and wasn't particularly good at catching, but he could throw well. He was also a good little hitter. I walked out into the backyard one afternoon just in time to watch him smack the ball over the backyard fence. He did it several times that summer, and we were always happy to retrieve it from the neighbor's yard. It continued to give us hope.

I was beginning to believe that our situation—physically, educationally, and emotionally—was starting to come together. Jackson had been accepted into the preschool that I thought would be most advantageous for his development, and he would receive services at our home elementary school, which would even better prepare him for kindergarten. Although I could never take my eyes off any ball I had in the air, I knew that all the effort that Bill and I were putting into Jackson's recovery, along with those of every teacher, therapist, and physician, was paying off. Abby was developing typically, and, albeit slowly, Jackson was recovering.

****

I still longed for alone time for myself and quality time with William—we were both ready to collapse. We wanted a week at our own camp.

Over the years, some colleagues questioned why I didn't have more of a backlog of vacation days in my leave bank. Working mothers with children with developmental differences use their vacation time for all-day doctors' appointments, therapy evaluations, school visits, and other programs related to their child's needs. I would have appreciated using more of those vacation days for actual vacation. Looking back, I realize that a day, or even half day, here and there dedicated to refortifying myself would have helped all of us.

Although Bill's and my relationship is solid, the sheer exhaustion of working full-time, keeping up with a home, and caring for two children (one with special needs) took its toll on us emotionally and physically. We no longer had the time or energy to be as supportive of each other as we once were, which did lead to a breakdown in communication on several fronts, mostly about child rearing and what was best for both children. But we were also not as open about our feelings for each other as we once were.

We turned inward and retreated to our own places of peace and calm, when we could find them, at the exclusion of the other. The impact of a special-needs child on a marriage or partnership can have both positive and negative effects, as Laura Marshak and Fran Pollock Prezant say in *Married with Special-Needs Children: A Couples' Guide to Keeping Connected:*

> The question about the impact of a child's disability on marriage cannot be answered by a single equation or formula. But some points are clear:
>
> - …Overall, you can think of having a child with a disability as amplifying what occurs in a more typical family and marriage. Closeness may be stronger, divisions greater, anger intensified, sadness deeper, parenting decisions weightier, and happy times more exhilarating.
> - There is no doubt that marriage is more complicated.
> - „Both in childrearing and marriage, having children with disabilities requires that we develop even better skills then others may need to have.[1]

Over time, Bill's and my experience as a couple would prove what I had read in *Married with Special-Needs Children* to be true: "We cannot lose sight of the fact that the lives of other family members also count. Each life is valuable and important. I believe in devotion and self-sacrifice but not to the point of entire negation of self or marriage."[2] Most people who haven't raised a child with learning or physical differences can't realize the strain it puts on a relationship. Kate Strohm went on to say in *Being the Other One*:

> It isn't so easy to function with strength and optimism. The day to day juggling of appointments and activities with a wide range of care providers can be exhausting and puts considerable strain on family functioning. It can be difficult for family members to interact positively with others when each feels pulled in so many different directions. There might be a breakdown in communication and the ability to support each other. The whole family system can become out of synch.[3]

We had been through a life-threatening circumstance, but we seemed to be moving beyond that acute phase of Jackson's illness. As we moved forward, it was time to focus more on our relationship. Babysitters were rare, because I didn't trust anyone with Jackson's medication other than the nanny, and she already worked for us more than forty hours a week. We took to at-home date nights after the kids went to bed, with dinner and a movie. We usually were too tired to make it through an entire movie and would finish it the next morning or evening, but our time together was vital.

CHAPTER 8

THE WORLD DOESN'T STOP FOR YOU

· · · · · · · · · · ·

Regardless of our own life events—a wedding, the birth of a child, an illness—life continues to go on around you. It doesn't stop, regardless of your needs. As Bill and I began to focus more attention on us, my parents' time together would come to an end.

The story of how they met could be the content of a movie script. It was in France, during World War II. My father was a US Air Force fighter pilot, and my mother was with the American Red Cross.

Before the war, my mother had been an elementary school teacher, principal, and later superintendent of a small school system. In her words, she "joined the Red Cross to go where the action was." I always interpreted that as "where the men were." She was assigned to my father's fighter squadron in Vitry-Le-Francois, where they met in a mess tent. They had their first date on New Year's Eve 1944 and were married eight months later in August 1945.

At almost ninety, my mother had experienced deteriorating health for about a year. I found with both of my parents that the tipping point for the decline in their physical health was about eighty-eight. My father, a year and a half younger than my mother, insisted he would care for her in their own home with the help of a home health aide. After all, as he said to me many times, "It's what you sign up for."

Two of my siblings and I were local and spent as much time helping him as we could. I say local, but my parents' house was about an hour away from Bill and me. I probably went over to their house about twice a month on the weekends. Between taking care of Jackson and Abby, working full-time, and trying to help my parents, my plate was overflowing. My mother's decline added a different emotional challenge to the mix already in my heart, as well as another logistical variable. When I was with my mother on weekends, I was worrying about Jackson and Abby, who already got very little of my time. When I was home on the weekends with my children, I worried about my mother. I knew my time with her would be limited, and I wanted to be with her.

My sister and brother seemed to have more time to offer, but their plates were full as well. My mother and I mostly talked about Jackson and Abby; babies and children had always been her favorite subject, and, given her background in education, she was especially interested in the pre-K program Jackson was attending. In addition, one of her neighbors had a degree in early childhood development and had previously taught at National Child Research Center, where Jackson would attend pre-K.

NCRC follows a model I think should be implemented in every school, worldwide. According to its website:

> A highly trained, multi-disciplinary faculty employs developmentally appropriate practices, supported by ongoing professional development and sound research. Essential to its role as a model of early childhood education is the creation of a diverse, respectful community. Both within and beyond the school community,

NCRC seeks opportunities to advocate for all children and their families.[1]

This was such a pivotal year for Jackson in so many ways. He had two teachers and an aide in a classroom of about twenty children, and he participated in speech and occupational therapy. The school also had a special education coordinator who kept close tabs on all the children with learning differences, and Jackson's teachers incorporated the learning strategies from the public school system's IEP.

The teachers also went on to apply their own progress summary for Jackson. It included strengthening his communication, self-help and functional skills, cognitive ability, social and emotional development, and physical development, including fine and gross motor skills. Meeting with NCRC to determine Jackson's goals for the year was night and day from the public school meetings. We sat in the classroom with Jackson's teachers and discussed his needs. There were no administrators, no psychologists, and no one who wouldn't be working closely with Jackson.

If any of the other families with children in the class knew Jackson was one of the children with different learning needs, Bill and I were not aware of it. As per the school's policy, the staff never indicated that Jackson was a child with learning differences, and I didn't say anything about his illness to other parents. The NCRC website stated:

> NCRC has a decades-long commitment to the inclusion of all children. NCRC welcomes children with mild to moderate special needs. Our goal is to collaborate with our families to make a positive difference in every child's educational experience. An inclusive school

> community broadens each child's perspective
> and brings added gifts to the program.[2]

I knew this would be a critical year for Jackson; it was a bridge from being in a preschool program for children with learning differences to being mainstreamed in a typical kindergarten classroom. His medical and developmental progress over the year would predict how successful he might be in a typical public kindergarten classroom. Bill and I were cautiously optimistic, but I didn't take my eyes off him throughout the year. Jackson's teachers were on top of all the Rainbows; I loved volunteering in the classroom just to observe the teaching model and watch Jackson's progress. Jackson was always happy to see me there, and I was happy to be there.

We implemented the services for special education, speech, and occupational therapy that Jackson had been given at our home elementary school. To help him transition, I went with him to the first few sessions for speech and OT. The therapists were very much in tune to Jackson's needs. Although I kept up with his progress, I never felt the need to attend a session with him that year, unless I was asked. Jackson went happily to every program; he was eager to learn and please and worked incredibly hard for his five little years.

It was time to test Jackson again to see where we were biochemically. He was catching up with his peers and continuing to develop and gain strength, but he was still delayed and far from being as healthy as we would like. He continued to tire easily, and his speech, fine motor skills, and overall well-being were still of concern.

The microbial panel continued to show elevated levels of yeast and once again showed slightly elevated levels of clostridia and *C. difficile*. We continued to treat the yeast, and Dr. Roberts added an additional probiotic that contained twenty billion cells of lactobacillus acidophilus daily, to fight the clostridia. Bill and I remained vigilant in ensuring that Jackson got every needed supplement every day. I constantly reminded myself that if I let up in any way, he could end up right back where we started. Never letting up took an immense amount of energy and sustained a constant level of stress that carried through all aspects of our lives.

Between work, normal household chores, two children, therapists, doctors, camps, school, and financial demands, we had such a structured and time-consuming routine that we rarely went out or saw friends. We weren't unhappy, just committed. This was life as we knew it for the time being, and I knew that true friends would understand that this was a very intense time in our lives. Inevitably, though, some friends that I sincerely enjoyed spending time with or talking to over the phone fell by the wayside.

We also used to exercise together. Bill still got an occasional run in but not with any regularity, and I wasn't doing anything to try to stay fit. It's very hard to find the motivation to exercise when you're constantly running on empty. There were many times when I think Bill and I felt like running away. We both needed short breaks, but we would always want to come home. I can't count the number of mornings I left for work and wanted to turn to the east and head for the beach—just two or three days by myself soaking up the energy of the warm sand, the ocean, and the sun. Instead, I settled for hot soaks in the bathtub, typically accompanied by Abby and a set of plastic Disney princesses. We spent many nights playing mermaid in the bathtub with those princesses.

******

The Saturday night before Thanksgiving, I got a call from my father, telling me that two days earlier my mother had slipped off the edge of her bed and fallen to the floor. She claimed to be fine, wasn't in any pain, and refused to be taken to the emergency room. She had a huge bruise on her forehead where she had hit the nightstand on her way down. My sister was there on Saturday morning, and after seeing how my mother looked, she suggested to my father that, regardless of my mother's refusal, she needed to be seen by a doctor. They dialed 911, and my mother was taken by ambulance to the emergency room of the local hospital. Given her frailty at that point, that was the only way she could be transported.

The bruise on her forehead was nothing, but an ultrasound showed that she had ruptured her small intestine when she fell. Because she wasn't in any pain and didn't have a fever, I knew her body was too weak to fight the infection in her abdomen. The doctors gave my father two options: they could give her high doses of antibiotics and see if she was any better by Sunday, or they would need to operate to repair her intestine. Without saying it, my father and I both knew she couldn't survive the infection, nor would she be able to survive surgery. He opted to start with the antibiotics.

I was in the middle of the budget season at work, the busiest time of year for me. I got up at five o'clock that Sunday morning and went to my office to finish the first review of the budgets for which I was responsible. I knew I would be out all week should my mother's life come to an end, and if I could get the first review done, it would give those who had submitted the budgets time to edit them while I was away. I got to the hospital at about four that afternoon. The antibiotics had helped but not enough to make a difference, and my mother was scheduled for surgery at five thirty.

Mom was awake and somewhat lucid when I arrived. I showed her pictures of Jackson and Abby, and we chatted briefly. My mother rarely handed out compliments to her daughters freely, at least not to me—but her last words to me were: "Ellen, you look so pretty today." By five o'clock, she had slipped into a coma from septic shock. We thought she had dozed off, but when the nurses came to check her vital signs, she was unresponsive.

My mother had a Do Not Resuscitate (DNR) order, so the nurses made her more comfortable in her bed and with doctor's orders gave her additional morphine, so she wouldn't struggle or suffer. My father sat on one side of the bed and held her hand, while my brother, sister, and I took turns holding the other and saying all the things we wanted to say to her. We left my father alone with her for a brief period, so he could have a private goodbye with his partner of more than sixty years.

I was fortunate enough to be holding my mother's hand when she died. I looked at the clock when she stopped breathing. It was five minutes after six on November 20, 2005. There's something very cathartic about holding the hand of the woman who gave you life when she takes her last breath, and I will always be grateful I was there. It was one of the most profound moments of my life. I never loved my mother more than I did at that moment, and she was gone. I would never be able to see her, talk to her, or touch her again in the same way I had for so many years.

I needed my mother as I plodded through the darkness of Jackson's recovery, and I started to miss her the minute she died. A friend of mine had read a piece at her own mother's funeral that resonated with me now more than ever.

Your mother is always with you. She is the whisper of the leaves as you walk down the street.

She's the smell of certain foods you remember, flowers you pick, the fragrance of life itself. She's the cool hand on your brow when you're not feeling well. She's your breath in the air on a cold winter's day. She is the sound of the rain that lulls you to sleep, the colors of a rainbow, she is Christmas morning. Your mother lives inside your laughter. She's the place you came from, your first home, and she's the map you follow with every step you take. She's your first love, your first friend, even your first enemy, but nothing on earth can separate you, not time, not space ... not even death. (Author unknown)

We took my father home, and by the time I got back to my house, it was around eleven o'clock. Bill had a fire in the fireplace for me, and I sat and stared into the flames. In their book *On Grief and Grieving*, Elisabeth Kubler-Ross and David Kessler write:

Everyone experiences many losses throughout life, but the death of a loved one is unmatched for its emptiness and profound sadness. Your world stops. You know the exact time your loved one died—or the exact moment you were told. It is marked in your mind. Your world takes on slowness, a surrealness. It seems strange that the clocks in the world continue when your inner clock does not ... Your loss and the grief that accompanies it are very personal, different from anyone else's. Others may share the experience of their losses. They may try to console you in the only way they know. But your loss stands alone in its meaning to you, in its painful uniqueness.[3]

My mother's death was the first that I had experienced of someone so close to me, and I was surprised to feel somewhat of a sense of relief after she died. I was grateful that she was no longer suffering. She had lived a long, full life, and there was no tragedy surrounding her death, but there was an overwhelming sense of sadness: "The relief and sadness mix together in a situation that has no resolve. When this occurs, your relief is the recognition that the suffering has ended, the pain is over, the disease no longer lives. Our loved one no longer has that illness, that disease. It has stopped causing her pain."[4]

There have been countless times that I've wanted to pick up the phone and call my mother since her death, usually to share my enthusiasm over a developmental or medical milestone that either Jackson or Abby reached.

My mother died on the Sunday before Thanksgiving. NCRC was an amazingly happy place, and the school had planned a celebration for the Rainbows that Tuesday. I wasn't in much of a celebratory mood, but I knew, had it been she, my mother would have been there. I had to tell the school that Jackson's grandmother had died, so they would be aware in case he brought it up, and the word had gotten out to some of the other parents in the class.

I knew I could hold it together at the party if no one offered too much compassion or sympathy. A few did, but I was okay until I saw a few sets of grandparents there. It struck me that my children had lost their grandmother at the very young ages of three and five years old. Jackson can still remember his grandmother, but Abby has no recollection of her.

While our mothers are alive, I think most women could write a book about the mistakes we perceive our mothers made in raising us, the times she embarrassed us, or her illogical reasoning. I only remember my mother now for the wonderful things that she was and did: all the birthdays and Christmases she made so special; the late-night talks when I'd broken up with a boyfriend or I didn't have a date for a dance; her incredible sense of beauty as seen through her garden, love of music, and selection of literature; and her being one of the first at the hospital to hold Jackson and Abby after they were born.

I will never forget the several occasions when I found my mother, in the middle of the night, looking out a window watching the quiet beauty and stillness of falling snow, and it was somehow fitting that a light snow fell throughout her entire memorial service. The service was on December 15, 2005. She would have been ninety on the eighteenth and had been looking forward to the party she would never physically attend. My mother loved pink champagne, and my family raised a glass and sang "Happy Birthday" to her in celebration of her life, her marriage, and her fifty-nine years of parenting.

During the holiday season, the parents of the children at NCRC received a gift of words from Susan Piggot, the director of the school, now retired, and a highly accomplished and amazing woman in her own right. Because my mother, who was my biggest fan and the one person I talked to most about parenting, was gone, Susan's words were especially meaningful to me, and continue to be:

> My holiday gift message to you: You are great parents. You are not perfect (and that's a good thing). You are doing the best you can every day, and some days are easier than others. Your children absolutely know that you love them, even when you are upset or impatient.

Being a parent is the hardest job in the world. Children don't come with a set of directions or a guarantee.

They all have special needs of one kind or another. They can be delightfully simple one minute and breathtakingly complex the next. You can love them so much that it hurts and want to kill them at the same time. Give yourself permission to lighten up. Don't try so hard. Less is more. Families are messy. And love conquers all.

I've had the little piece of paper on which these words are written in my wallet since Jackson was five. I take them out periodically to read and remind myself that, most of the time, I am the mother I want to be.

CHAPTER 9

PROGRESS

. . . .

That January in pre-K, Jackson had developed one of the worst ear infections he had ever had. He missed a full week of school, with a fever of 103 degrees for four days. On the third day, as I was trying to get him to eat something, he sat up in bed and with a pitiful little voice said, "Mommy, I think I'm feeling better today." He really wasn't. But I've never known a child with such a resilient and positive attitude.

He was back on antibiotics, accompanied by a regression. He typically became lethargic, irritable, and somewhat less verbal; wouldn't feed himself; and wanted to be held. Dr. Roberts suggested that the next time he required an antibiotic, we would give him the antifungal Nystatin along with it, to see if we could avoid another temporary setback. He recovered after about two weeks and was back in school. I hoped it would be some time before we got the opportunity to test the Nystatin theory.

For some reason, I was home on a school day in February and was able to take Jackson to NCRC. The school was in a large, old Victorian house in the middle of a beautiful neighborhood. Jackson and I got as far as the front porch, and he refused to go inside. I tried to reason with him, cajole him, and even physically force him, but he cried and dug in further. He had never behaved this way, except for the first two days I took him to summer camp. Because I spent time in his classroom and came and went without him clinging to me, I didn't think this was about separation anxiety; besides, he was getting too old for that.

I could see Susan in her office from the porch and was able to get her attention. She came to help, and I told her Jackson didn't want to go to school that day. Susan immediately went and got Katie, the special education coordinator, for me. Katie quite skillfully had Jackson in her office playing with a toy in about two minutes, and up to the Rainbow classroom within five.

I always attributed moments like this to how Jackson was feeling at any particular time, thinking he may have been experiencing the residual effect of the recent illness and course of antibiotics. He was in such capable hands at NCRC. The administrators, teachers, and special educators will never know how grateful I will always be for that year. It was a year of growth and recovery, not only for Jackson but for Bill, Abby, and me as well.

Contributing to my own growth and knowledge that year, the school regularly conducted parent-education classes. I attended several discussions with child psychologists about children's behavior and with special education advocates, like Suzie, about how to advocate for your child within the school system. There were also discussions with nutritionists about how different foods affect a child's brain and development. In addition, the parents organized potluck dinners, so we could become better acquainted with the other families of children in the class.

I almost proved myself an unfit mother to a five-year-old when, at the first dinner, I announced that Jackson's favorite movie was *Alien.* They all looked at me as if I was out of my mind—even Bill. He finally came to my rescue and announced to the others, "She means *ET!*" Jackson had fallen in love with *ET* that year, but he called it *Alien.* We had gotten so used to calling the movie *Alien* at home that I just absentmindedly blurted it out. Big difference between an R-rated horror film and a sweet PG-rated movie about a lovable extraterrestrial.

Despite such occasional blunders, and because the school wasn't very far from my office, the teachers and parents welcomed me. About once a month during lunchtime, I'd go to read to the Rainbows. I think they were the cutest group of children I've seen in any one classroom. Their theme song was "The Rainbow Connection" by Paul Williams, and they sang it at every opportunity. I laughed every time I heard those little four and five-year-olds sing, "Someday we'll find it, the rainbow connection, the lovers, the dreamers, and me." I don't think any of them ever questioned what a lover or a dreamer was; they just sang their song with great enthusiasm.

Spring was approaching, and we started thinking about sports and physical activity again. Both children had taken gymnastics over the winter, which they loved, and Abby had tried ballet, until the nanny told me she was probably better off in gymnastics. Apparently, the ballet teacher wanted the class to pretend they were butterflies, and Abby had told her she'd prefer to gallop like a horse. Based on Jackson's assessment from his last summer camp, we decided to put him in T-ball. He could already hit the ball with consistency, and we thought it would be a better experience than soccer had been. Bill signed him up, and off they went.

It wasn't the disaster that soccer had been, but Jackson still didn't like it; there was a lot of standing around, and he was mostly bored. He was able to play the full season, however. I took him to a game one weekend when Bill was out of town. Jackson was playing third base, and I watched as several children hit the ball and ran the bases backward, let the ball roll between their legs, and ran into each other, knocking each other down trying to catch the ball. Not many runners ever made it to third base. About thirty-five minutes into the game, Jackson yelled to me from his position, "Mom, can we go home now?"

"We need to stay and finish the game," I told him. He sneered slightly, but he stayed on third base and made it through the end of the game.

****

That spring, as I continued to search the internet for new information on leaky gut, I stumbled upon the Specific Carbohydrate Diet and, at the time, found an article on the website for the Children's Neurobiological Solutions Foundation. The article, "A Diet to Satiate the Brain and Calm the Tummy: Benefits of the Specific Carbohydrate Diet," grabbed my attention. The second paragraph in the article indicated that:

> Focused on more obvious cognitive or motor skill issues, many parents and physicians may not make the connection between their child's neurological disorder with their gastrointestinal symptoms, or vice versa. However, more and more parents and clinicians are beginning to connect these two nervous systems, the Central Nervous System and the Enteric Nervous System, and are finding that correcting digestive imbalances can lead to significant overall improvement in their child's mental and physical health and in several cases reduce or even eliminate seizure activity.

The article went on to explain leaky gut syndrome and how diet can provide an intervention to this vicious cycle by depriving intestinal microbes of their energy source while providing excellent nutrition to the patient.

The SCD is a strict grain-free, lactose-free, and sucrose-free dietary regimen intended for those suffering from Crohn's disease, ulcerative colitis, celiac disease, IBD, and IBS. The diet is based on the principle that specifically selected carbohydrates requiring minimal digestion are well absorbed, leaving virtually nothing for intestinal microbes to feed on.

Some families had found that one or two years on the diet had been enough to thoroughly heal their child's intestine to the point that the child could return to a normal diet without side effects. Was this a find or what? Despite the amazing medical team we had working with us, I was still searching for anything we might have missed or any new information that might be available.

I didn't make a move with regard to Jackson's care without consulting Dr. Roberts. I called her, saying I'd found "the cure" for Jackson. She didn't exactly stop me in my tracks, but she explained that it might be a good idea to go completely gluten- and casein-free before we went directly with the Specific Carbohydrate Diet. Eliminating gluten and casein would be difficult enough without going straight to the SCD. We would wait to talk to a nutritionist about diet.

In addition, Dr. Roberts ordered lab work to test for heavy metals—the one test we had not yet done. This test requires hair samples. Jackson had always had a short haircut, so the test was delayed while we let his hair grow long enough to get a decent sample. As I recall, it had to be at least one inch long and cut close to the scalp. I sat Jackson up in a chair and cut small chunks of hair from all over the back of his head. When I was done, it looked like Edward Scissorhands had given him a haircut.

The test results showed he had elevated levels of aluminum, mercury, tin, and iodine, yet he was low in sodium, potassium, manganese, boron, and lithium. His copper level was normal, which was little consolation given the imbalance of everything else. The common symptoms associated with all the high indicators included fatigue, poor memory and cognitive dysfunction, neuromuscular disorders, GI tract irritation, muscle weakness, and hypersensitivity reactions of the immune or other systems. The lab results also indicated that "hair aluminum is commonly elevated in children and adults with low zinc and behavioral/learning disorders such as ADD, ADHD, and autism."

We didn't think Jackson was being exposed to high levels of aluminum, mercury, tin, or iodine. What we concluded was that Jackson wasn't clearing normal amounts of these elements from his system the way a healthy individual might, and that was probably due to other imbalances in his system.

We are all exposed to some level of these metals on a regular basis from cooking with aluminum, eating anything canned, eating fish that are commonly higher in mercury, using aluminum foil, and so on. The difference is that a system that hasn't been compromised can typically clear them on its own. Dr. Roberts referred us to a well-known and highly credentialed nutritionist.

My first appointment with the nutritionist was in early July, and her reputation for being brilliant had preceded her. Her credentials alone were good enough for me, but I also liked the way her website, at the time, described her practice:

> Dana Laake Nutrition provides preventive and therapeutic nutritional services. We welcome patients of all ages from prenatal through the

elder population. Working in partnership with patients and their healthcare professionals, we utilize an individualized approach in evaluation and treatment. Our recommendations address the specific goals of each patient and are based on medical history, family history, conditions, lifestyle, medications, diet, supplementation, physical evaluation, and laboratory testing. Each patient is expected to maintain a primary care provider and specialty care where indicated. Our goal is to complement other healthcare being provided.[1]

I had never seen a nutritionist before and didn't really know what to expect. After four hours with the woman, I thought my head would explode. My brain hurt. I don't think I've ever tried to absorb so much information in four hours in my life. Dana was so brilliantly knowledgeable that I must admit it was a little overwhelming. I was taking notes as fast as I could, while she was keying into her computer. I finally asked if she was typing everything she was telling me. Of course, she was doing just that, and she would give me a copy of everything she was recommending before I left.

My notes said that we would start a trial of a gluten-and casein-free diet. We would not go straight to a Specific Carbohydrate Diet, but Dana did give me a modified version of the SCD. Dr. Roberts had sent her Jackson's test results. Dana focused on the low magnesium, indicating that it can cause both attention deficit and the ability to hyper focus. It can also lead to muscle spasms (myoclonus), impulsivity, and sensory and mood issues. She indicated that we needed to also add more protein to each of Jackson's meals and that instead of giving him fruit juice, we should give him seltzer water with just enough juice to flavor it, along with fruit popsicles and blueberries.

She went into the chemistry of everything Jackson needed— and that's when my brain started to hurt. Jackson would need a mineral supplement compounded with magnesium glycinate, L-taurine, potassium, zinc, vitamin B5, biotin, and lithium orotate (a naturally occurring food source micronutrient mineral). He would also need a B complex vitamin supplement to include P-5-P, B complex, B12, R-5-P, more B5, CoQ10, and L-carnitine. I had no clue what half of these things did— and had never heard of P-5-P or R-5-P—but whatever they were, Dana thought Jackson would benefit from them. She also explained that nutrients are regulated by the body so that when there is deficiency, absorption and retention increase. When nutrient levels are sufficient, absorption and retention decline. It is called homeostasis (balance) and the reasons supplements have such a high safety level, as compared to medications, which are metabolized by the body and not subject to the homeostasis effect.

I researched them to find that P-5-P is a form of vitamin B6, and R-5-P stands for ribose 5-phosphate and is an enzyme that plays an important role in ribose metabolism. Ribose is a type of sugar normally made in the body from glucose. Ribose plays important roles in the synthesis of RNA, DNA, and the energy-containing substance adenosine triphosphate (ATP). This was all about as clear as mud to me; I was in way over my head.

Dana faxed the prescriptions for the compounds to a formulating pharmacy, gave me a packet of information that was extremely helpful but would take me months to digest, and sent me on my way. I had taken the morning off from work and had to go back to my office. I would have called in sick, gone home, and pulled my covers over my head, but I had a strategic planning exercise that afternoon and had to be there. I got a grip on myself and headed to work.

The meeting was with my immediate boss and two close colleagues. They asked how the morning had gone, and I burst into tears. My son was now, officially, a gluten- and casein-free chemistry experiment, and I would spend my free time shopping in five different grocery stores instead of the two that I typically used. Jackson was a terribly picky eater. How could I ever be successful at a gluten- and dairy-free diet? What if I couldn't find enough variety for him to eat? And I knew he would never drink seltzer water flavored with fruit juice; he'd want the real thing.

I was trying very hard to maintain some level of internal emotional balance, but adding the new variable of nutritional imbalance was making it increasingly difficult. I regularly thought of leaving my job and staying home with my children, but it wasn't financially feasible; supplements, speech, OT, doctor visits, special camps, and a year of private pre-K all adds up to a lot of money. Even with giving up our full-time nanny, we couldn't afford it.

I called my most experienced resource and friend, Megan, that night. She assured me I could do this. She also had a child on a gluten-free diet and could recommend gluten-free breads, muffins, pasta, and bagels she had found through her own trial and error. She was still searching for a dairy-free cheese that wasn't tasteless and didn't have the consistency of rubber.

Megan told me the basics I would need to get started. I went out the next weekend to explore the world of mostly organic markets that had a decent selection of gluten- and dairy-free foods. With the press that celiac disease has gotten, and with so many children with autism benefiting from a gluten- and dairy-free diet, there are significantly more good products on the market today than there were even five years ago, though they continue to be excessively expensive.

Two days after I saw Dana, Jackson had an appointment with the neurologist. He had ordered an EEG, which would show Jackson's current brain wave pattern. In addition, he had ordered blood work that would show the level of Lamictal in Jackson's system at peak and trough levels, and he would have the results for us during our visit.

We hadn't changed the Lamictal dose since Jackson had become stable on the medication, just after his third birthday. He'd been taking it for three years, and we suspected, given his physical and metabolic growth, that he may no longer be at a therapeutic level. This meant he was potentially outgrowing the dose he was on and weaning himself off the medication. We would complete the EEG in the morning, go out to lunch, and return to see the doctor in the afternoon. This was a typical routine when we had an EEG, as it gave the neurology team time to interpret the test before our afternoon appointment.

Jackson's behavior was flawless during the EEG. He did everything the tech asked him to do. The neurology assessment and clinic notes from Dr. Billy affirmed our thoughts.

Clinic Notes
Jackson has done extremely well. The EEG done today in our lab showed some clinical unresponsiveness during hyperventilation, but no true seizure activity. No spikes or abnormalities noted ... This information leads me to conclude that it is reasonable to try slowly tapering the Lamictal once Dr. Roberts is done making whatever metabolic adjustments she wants to make. Jackson's mother will let me know when the metabolic issues are worked out and I will set up a tapering schedule for Lamictal. Follow-up will be here in six months.

> Jackson has grown a tremendous amount since his last visit ... his use of language is markedly improved. I asked him what he did yesterday at the pool and he said, "jumped off the diving board and put my face in the water."
>
> He makes very good eye contact. He is happy and bright. He continues to do nicely and will enter regular kindergarten in the fall. His sleep pattern is stabilized. His behavioral profile is essentially normal ... At his last visit, mother was concerned about some unusual myoclonic jerks while falling asleep, but she now realizes that those are not seizure activity but are likely physiologic myoclonus in sleep ...

Jackson's visit with the neurologist was actually fun. They had a great conversation about how he liked to spend his time and what he was doing in camp. I was almost giddy with the results of the EEG and the fact that it might be time to wean Jackson off the seizure meds. The Lamictal level was 4.8 at peak and 3.8 at trough; a therapeutic level is between 4 and 18. Could this horrible aspect of Jackson's illness be almost behind us?

Under the watchful eyes of Dana and Dr. Roberts, I introduced the supplements slowly over several weeks. We also transitioned Jackson to a gluten- and dairy-free diet. Between the supplements and the diet, Jackson's overall well-being, mood, attention span, and ability to process language improved almost immediately. His eyes were brighter; he was happy, less irritable, and was far from starving to death on his new diet. We decided not to change too many variables at one time and let Jackson have more time on the supplements before we started to taper the seizure meds.

****

It was the end of the school year, and assessments and reviews were starting to roll in. We were developing new OT goals for Jackson. He had done well in achieving goals dealing with motor planning and with what's called "constructional praxis," a task requiring three-dimensional manipulation. His private OT, Christine, added the goals of pumping his legs on a swing with good timing and rhythm and completing five monkey bars independently, which he would work on over the summer.

Jackson was not doing as well with fine motor and visual perceptual motor skill development and had mastered only one goal in that area. Yet Christine added additional goals: tossing and catching a tennis ball with one hand, tossing objects at a target with increased accuracy, and holding a pencil with consistent wrist extension and precise opposition of thumb and fingers, or tripod grasp.

The end-of-year notes suggested that Jackson should continue to be seen weekly. They advised that Jackson "be seen by an ophthalmologist and or a developmental optometrist to rule out problems with a) visual acuity (resolving power of the eye or sight) and b) vision (the use of the information gathered from the eye such as binocular fusion, tracking, visual motor processing). If in fact Jackson is experiencing visual deficits, this may also affect his attention, focus, and visual motor abilities."

Working with the school speech pathologist, Jennifer had also updated goals for Jackson that would be used both within the school system and privately. Again, they were all about receptive and expressive language skills. Jackson had never had an articulation problem, but he sometimes struggled to find the right words. The new goals addressed following directions, understanding quantity and time concepts, recalling details from a story, logically answering questions, using correct pronouns, retelling a short story, and defining words with appropriate detail. Some of these goals were the same as they had always been, except now they were at a more difficult level. When Jackson started preschool, he had been working on following one- or two-step directions; now he was working on following complex directions.

Bill and I were encouraged by Jackson's progress, but we still weren't sure he was ready for a typical kindergarten classroom. It was true that his development during the year at NCRC had been astounding. His teachers commented:

> With Jackson's impressive social growth in the classroom, we are seeing a boon in social language with peers, good eye contact, and new scripts and roles for play. This level of sustained interaction with peers is having a wonderfully positive impact on his communication and cognitive development.

> We are thrilled with Jackson's success as we watch him laughing with his buddies and talking up a storm, their arms linked. This is what we wanted for Jackson this year! … His charming, endearing personality, loving nature, and great perseverance make Jackson a wonderfully rich and complex little boy. He is a unique individual who contributes a tremendous amount to our classroom. We will miss him dearly and wish Jackson and his family all the best next year.

With comments like these, we remained cautiously optimistic that Jackson would be successful in a mainstreamed kindergarten environment. I spoke with the resource teacher he had been seeing at our home elementary school to get her opinion and advice about school placement for kindergarten. She felt that Jackson was ready but suggested that I speak with the L&D teacher whose class Jackson would attend should he not be mainstreamed. Once the L&D teacher listened to Jackson's history and the progress he had made, she was adamant he be placed in a typical kindergarten classroom. He was making great progress and needed to be in with his typical peers to continue developing as he had at NCRC.

The decision was made. Jackson would attend kindergarten at our home elementary school and would even have another NCRC Rainbow in his classroom with him. I reluctantly said goodbye to NCRC, the staff, and Jackson's wonderful teachers. How I wished they had a kindergarten classroom for him. One more year there would have given me such confidence in Jackson's foundational development. They did have one higher level of preschool, but Jackson would be six in a few weeks; he needed a kindergarten program.

That year, Jackson had progressed not only cognitively but developmentally. For the first time, Jackson had been invited to birthday parties, playdates, and other social events. We invited all the Rainbows to Jackson's sixth birthday. It was the first year where we could invite a group of school friends, as opposed to family or close personal friends. We had invited the kids and their parents to a children's splash park run by the county parks department.

The morning started off cool and cloudy, and we were concerned that no one would show up. In fact, almost all the Rainbows came, and we had the park to ourselves. The kids spent hours running in and out of fountains, through waterfalls into caves, standing under buckets that would dump water on them without notice, and climbing on elephants and other animals that suddenly spewed water in some form or fashion. Jackson was finally well enough to enjoy life again. He was a completely different child from the one who, just three years earlier, could only sit and stare at the television. He had the time of his life that day.

Jackson's condition seemed to become more chronic as opposed to acute, and we saw the same kinds of growth that he had achieved in the prior year when he returned to speech and language camp during the summer break. The theme that summer was sports. The first week was about exercise and nutrition, then basketball, track and field, soccer, and baseball. He was enthusiastic about camp that year, and he never had an issue with my leaving him.

Jackson had developed such remarkably stronger social skills during his year at NCRC that he now loved to be around and play with other children. We took his bike to camp with him so that he could work on balance and consistent pedaling for those five weeks. He had ridden a two-wheeler for two years but had never felt confident enough to let us take the training wheels off. Christine was also working on biking with him when she saw him each week. Things were going well in many ways. But we didn't think we'd ever have the luxury of becoming complacent, and our bank account was reflective of our efforts.

Our insurance company had been paying their portion of Jackson's therapies and doctors' visits. As long as we provided the letters of medical necessity and proper documentation, we had very few problems. Just before Jackson's sixth birthday, we received a letter from the insurance company stating that Jackson had exceeded his lifetime benefits. Surely this was a mistake. He was five years old; how could he possibly have exceeded his lifetime benefits?

We have changed health plans multiple times since then. I don't have a record of what the dollar amount of those benefits were, but they were quite high. Today, according to the US. Department of Health and Human Services, under the Affordable Care Act, health plans are not allowed to place annual or lifetime dollar limits on most benefits you receive. "Under the current law, lifetime limits on most benefits are prohibited in any health plan or insurance policy. Previously, many plans set a lifetime limit — a dollar limit on what they would spend for your covered benefits during the entire time you were enrolled in that plan. You were required to pay the cost of all care exceeding those limits."[2]

We appealed their assessment. Every doctor had to write another letter of medical necessity, and Jennifer conducted and documented a comprehensive speech-language evaluation. At six, Jackson was nine months behind on expressive vocabulary and up to twenty-seven months behind on recalling sentences.

Between the doctors' letters and Jennifer's assessment, we won the appeal, and for the time being, the insurance company continued to cover Jackson's services. We found that insurance companies will look diligently at any treatment plan to find rationale to deny coverage. Bill put hours and hours into filing claims and communicating with our health insurance company. With the Affordable Care Act being threatened, I wonder what families with fewer resources of support will be able to do in a similar situation. Will their children have to go without care and the early intervention they need to develop?

Although Jackson would continue seeing Jennifer, it turned out that this was the last time he would attend speech and language camp. He had a great summer. He loved playing with the other children, he learned board games, and he continued to work on language processing and fine motor skills, like writing.

In her final notes, the director mentioned how very proud she was of the progress Jackson had made. To us, on a day-to-day basis, it seemed like Jackson's recovery was quite slow. But looked at from another perspective, it was clear he had made monumental progress over three years. His development was finally coming together, and I was beginning to have a good feeling about kindergarten.

CHAPTER 10

SEIZURE-FREE

• • • • • • • • • • •

As the African proverb goes, it takes a village to raise a child. In today's global world, most families' villages consist of parents, grandparents, teachers, pediatricians, clergy, friends, and so on. If you have a child with differences, your village may expand into several. It may include special caregivers, developmental pediatricians, neurologists, therapists—speech, occupational, physical, and psychological. Your child may also need special educators, nutritionists, geneticists, orthopedists, and a host of others.

Likewise, parents of a child with special needs require their own unique expanded village for support. A very wise and well-respected female mentor I know once said, "There are three variables that keep working parents balanced on their tightrope. One is their spouse or partner, another is their work supervisor, and the last is their child-care provider." If any one of these variables is disrupted, then that parent will stumble, if not completely fall off balance. We were about to experience stumbling firsthand.

Jackson had the same nanny since he was six months old. She was impeccable with infants, but I was learning that she didn't have the patience needed to care for an energetic preschooler and kindergartner. I found her losing her temper with the children more often and not allowing them to do the fun things little children love to do—play the piano, get dirty, exert their independence, and generally make as much noise as humanly possible. She liked everything in its place and the house quiet. She loved to sit and rock babies. But we were beyond that stage, and life at our house would only get worse for her, and for us. My patience was wearing thin with her, and hers with me.

About two weeks before Jackson started kindergarten, I came home from work one day to find him standing in a corner crying, with his arms held up over his head. I had no idea what he had done, but I suspected that the punishment had exceeded the crime. I asked the nanny why Jackson's arms were over his head.

"To make his arms hurt," she said.

"Tell him he can put his arms down," I said.

She gave me a nasty look, and I told her once again, "Tell him he can put his arms down."

She picked up her purse and walked out the front door, never acknowledging my request.

By the next afternoon, we had a mutual understanding that she would no longer be in our employment. I took another week of vacation days to take care of the kids while I tried to find and train a new nanny. I did two things differently this time. I went through a nanny agency, and I also went to a home health service. The agency I used was into quantity and not so much quality. I interviewed about ten women and felt comfortable with only two. I also interviewed several home health aides— and felt comfortable with none.

One potential home health aide did offer some helpful suggestions on how to better organize Jackson's medication— not my chart but the medication itself. The original nanny had been with us throughout the acute stage of Jackson's regression and had learned his medication along with Bill and me. I realized that giving Jackson all his medication and supplements could potentially be overwhelming for a new caregiver.

I organized all the medication and supplements as the home health aide suggested, which also made it easier for Bill and me to administer doses. I bought five pill dispensers and labeled them breakfast, lunch, afternoon snack, dinner, and bedtime. I started filling them once a week, to help prevent anyone from making a mistake with Jackson's meds, and dedicated an entire cabinet in our kitchen to the pill dispensers and bottles of supplements and medication. I also organized and labeled a shelf in the door of the refrigerator for all the supplements that needed to be refrigerated.

We interviewed one more candidate, whom Bill and I both immediately liked, and her references checked out glowingly. She was a wonderful woman, not at all intimidated by Jackson's medication chart or his history, and the children grew to love her. She stayed with us for the next two years until she and her husband would welcome twins of their own.

****

The first day of kindergarten was exciting and stressful. This was the first time Jackson would ride a bus by himself. It arrived right on time, and he hopped on happily. Like most mothers, my eyes filled with tears as I watched my little boy head out into the world on his own. I walked home, got in my car, beat the bus to school, and hid behind the side of the school building so he wouldn't see me. I watched his bus arrive and his teacher greet him as he got off, then saw him safely enter the building.

Just as I was leaving, the principal spotted me. It was a good thing he knew who I was, or I might have been arrested for stalking kindergarteners. On my way to work, I called Mary and told her what I had done. Her response was, "Of course you did. I followed every one of my children's buses to school on the first day of kindergarten and made sure they got into the building safely." She didn't, however, get out of her car and lurk in the schoolyard.

By the third day of kindergarten, Jackson had a fever of 102. I took him to the pediatrician and learned that Jackson had a strep infection for the first time. Obviously, he needed an antibiotic; we called Dr. Roberts and got the appropriate dose of Nystatin to keep yeast at bay, filled the prescription, then gave it to Jackson for three weeks and watched. There was no regression with the antibiotic. The Nystatin had done its job—another first. As soon as the strep was under control, Jackson was himself again. He was back in school but had missed half of his first week of kindergarten.

The teachers who worked with Jackson that year were just as dedicated as his teachers at NCRC had been. I met with them early in the year to explain Jackson's history, his therapies, and where we were in his recovery. After hearing the story, I think his kindergarten teacher was determined to help him succeed. From the beginning of the school year, I watched her engage every child in her classroom to ensure each one of them worked to their fullest potential in learning to read, understanding math concepts, continuing to develop social skills, and building the foundation they needed to move on to first grade.

Jackson's IEP for kindergarten indicated he needed help with receptive and expressive language processing, fine motor skills, ability to pay attention, and compliance with some tasks. The NCRC resource teacher had written in her progress update that "Jackson's area of need is his attention. He performs very well on tasks when he is focused. He often looks away when coloring and needs support from an adult to redirect him back to the task at hand."

Jackson didn't like to color, and frankly his drawing skills were abysmal, but I'm not sure he didn't come by them naturally. I have trouble drawing stick figures. Once, Bill drew a unicorn for Abby, who asked him if it was a hyena.

The IEP also documented that Jackson's strengths were his fluency of speech, speech intelligibility, and voice. He was strong in letter identification and letter sound awareness, and he had improved in writing numbers to ten and writing uppercase letters, cutting skills, matching numbers to quantity, and rote counting to twenty-nine—and he was eager to learn. Jackson was practicing telling simple stories, using correct prepositions and pronouns, and defining items.

The American Academy of Pediatrics books continued to be great resources for me in benchmarking Jackson's development outside of school and his IEP. I had purchased *Caring for Your School-Age Child, Ages 5 to 12* and referred to it regularly.

During the summer before kindergarten, Jackson had an additional OT assessment by the school system to see what, if any, services he would need during the school year. The same needs were identified that had been previously documented— pencil grasp, pressure in writing, and hand strength. This evaluation, as did Christine's, showed that Jackson scored below average in the developmental test of visual motor integration.

Increasingly over the past year, Jackson had been closing or covering his right eye, telling us his "eyes were fighting with each other." After speaking with Dr. Roberts, Bill and I decided to take him to a developmental optometrist for evaluation, as Jennifer, his speech pathologist, and Christine, his occupational therapist, had recommended earlier.

In addition to an interpretation of Jackson's needs, the eye doctor's assessment explained the role of a developmental optometrist.

During the early years of life when all of the senses become integrated, the visual mechanism becomes the primary sensory-motor system through which the child interacts with and learns about the world. Through time, experience, and maturation, the visual system develops higher-level functions that ultimately allow individuals to understand and utilize symbols for thinking and communication. One of the purposes of my developmental evaluation is to establish the degree to which the visual system has achieved this primary role.

The optometrist documented that Jackson's eyes were healthy and measured 20/20 for distance targets and almost perfect for near targets. However, his visual perceptual and thinking abilities were below his chronological age. The ultimate diagnosis was "developmental delays of Jackson's basic sensory integration foundation, visual developmental delays of approximately one-and-a-half years and probable mild binocular vision dysfunction (inadequate ability to sustain alignment of the eyes and fusion of the information received by the visual cortex from the eyes)." The optometrist recommended in his write-up that Jackson have vision therapy once a week for a year and therapeutic lenses, for indoor use only, that would foster the development of spatial awareness and orientation.

But in person, he told us that Jackson's needs were really borderline, that he wasn't sure the recommended therapies would help, and that Jackson could potentially outgrow the problem on his own. After significant discussion and debate, Bill and I opted to watch and wait. Jackson already had four therapy sessions a week after school, two each of OT and speech, and a demanding medication and supplements regimen. There was very little time left in his schedule for anything else.

We were barely keeping up financially with everything else we were doing for him, and we were starting to accrue some debt. I kept going back to the neurologist's words, "We're not going to break your bank account." It was hard not to when we could see Jackson's progress daily. Every penny we spent recovering him was well worth it.

Bill and I had asked the school for a ninety-day review after the start of kindergarten. We wanted the chance to speak with his teachers and therapists in a formal setting to see how he was doing in school and whether the IEP was appropriate. All working with him thought that he was doing great and mainstream kindergarten was the right fit; they recommended that the IEP be continued without any changes.

Kindergarten children in our county receive an "early childhood observational record" twice a year—essentially, their report card. The children are assessed against fifty-nine criteria. At the end of December, Jackson received thirty-nine I's—meaning he was "in process of developing the behavior or skill"—and twenty P's, indicating he was proficient and had "consistently demonstrated the behavior or skill." Jackson had either mastered or was working toward everything he was supposed to be able to do by the end of the school year. We still had another half year of kindergarten, during which he could potentially develop further.

I knew that for every year that went by, Jackson was not only catching up from the regression he had experienced but also was missing some of the development he should have been gaining, through all the years he was trying to recover. This is why it was important for Jackson's recovery that he be placed in a classroom with his typical peers. It would take several more years for him to be able to reach his chronological age. Despite that reality, we had a great deal to celebrate at Christmas. Abby was continuing to develop typically, and Jackson, albeit slowly, was catching up with his peers.

****

My father gave Jackson a magnetic dartboard for Christmas; they sat in his living room and played off and on for hours. My father was in his chair, while Jackson stood by his side, putting them at the same height, and I propped the dartboard up on a chair opposite them. It was a perfect setup for a six-year-old and almost ninety-year-old.

It had been just over a year since my mother died, and my father was lonely without her. I had had a quiet conversation with him the day after her death and suggested, not now but when he was ready, he might want to consider moving to a retirement community. It was going to get lonely in their house, and he might want more social interaction than he would have there alone.

"Ellen, it's already lonely," he had replied. I think that was the saddest thing my father ever said to me; my mother hadn't even been gone for twenty-four hours.

Two weeks after Christmas, on the morning of January 7, 2007, thirteen months after my mother died, I got a call from my sister to tell me our father had died in his sleep. We couldn't reach my brother, but we were able to leave a message for him to call us. I contacted my other two sisters and drove the hour to my father's house. I was a little surprised to find a police cruiser in front of the house, but apparently when someone dies alone at home, the police have to be notified, to rule out foul play. The police officer was very kind given the circumstances and, except for contacting the funeral home, took care of most details for us that day.

My father had kept the home health aide he had hired to help him with my mother. She came every day to help cook, do laundry, and basically check on him. He also had a good friend two doors down, who had told him after my mother died, "Joe, you have to call every day to let me know you're okay, and if I don't hear from you, I'll call you." It was a great arrangement having someone who cared so much for him in the neighborhood.

When the health aide left on January 6, Daddy told her to wake him up by nine o'clock when she came in the next morning, because he didn't want to sleep late. Annie arrived the next morning to find him in his bed with the TV still on from the night before. One of the neighbors said to me, "What ninety-year-old man doesn't want to die in his sleep with a remote control in his hand?" He must have fallen asleep watching the news, as he did most nights, but he never woke up to turn off the television.

My mother had wanted to be cremated, but my father didn't. We honored my mother's wishes and kept her urn until his death. Daddy had a few favorite shirts, one of which was a Hawaiian print that Mary and I had picked up for him on a trip to Maui. I washed it and a pair of slacks and took it to the funeral home. I was a little hesitant of what the funeral director might think of us burying my father in a Hawaiian print shirt, but it was his favorite, and we all wanted him to rest in comfort.

If I recall correctly, the funeral director's comment was: "The Hawaiian shirt's a nice touch." We put my mother's urn in the casket with my father, and we buried them together with full military honors. I found it remarkable that, after fighting in World War II, flying surveillance during the Korean War, and serving with the head of the Pacific Air Command during the conflict in Vietnam, not to mention raising five children, my father was able to die peacefully in his sleep. Although none of us were ready to let him go, one of my sisters was able to articulate, "Isn't this what we all wanted for him?"

I was struck by two realizations after my father died. Having been blessed with good parents, I learned that losing one parent is sad, but when the second is gone, the dimensions of your life shift dramatically. You are no longer someone's child, and you no longer have the unconditional love that only a parent can provide. The two people who were always on my side, no matter what, were gone. Elisabeth Kubler-Ross and David Kessler write in *On Grief and Grieving*:

> We are not accustomed to the emotional upheaval that accompanies a loss. People experience a wide array of emotions after a loss, from not caring to being on edge to feeling angry or sad about everything. We can go from feeling okay to feeling devastated in a minute without warning ... We can touch the pain directly for only so long until we have to back away ... If we did not go back and forth emotionally, we could never have the strength to find peace in our loss.[1]

In searching for peace in my loss, I found myself with an overwhelming sense of responsibility to instill in my own children the positive values my parents had instilled in me. Although still grieving, I was able to turn my attention back to Jackson and Abby.

******

For several months now, Jackson had been on the supplements that Dr. Roberts and Dana Laake had prescribed; he was stable, and he was showing marked improvement in his stamina, his ability to engage and stay engaged, and his overall well-being. He was less irritable and more cooperative. Six months had gone by since our last appointment with the neurologist, and it was time to talk to him again about taking Jackson off of seizure medication.

I made the appointment with trepidation—I didn't ever want to see anyone have a seizure again, especially not Jackson. Under the neurologist's direction, we started reducing the Lamictal by a small and consistent dose on a weekly basis. I spoke with everyone who had regular contact with Jackson—teachers, therapists, caregivers, and close family members—to explain the process of titrating medication and to ask that they look for any sign of change in behavior or potential seizure activity.

After eleven weeks of slowly reducing the medication, we stopped it completely. Jackson was off his medication, more alert, and free of any visible seizures. At the end of March 2007, the neurologist repeated the EEG. His summary report stated: "A normal EEG. There are no seizure discharges or lateralizing signs ..."

Jackson was discharged from his care. I wasn't sure I was ready to be discharged from his care, but we had finally cleared enough toxins from Jackson's system that his brain was no longer trying to clear them for him. It took me several months—almost a year—to grasp that this aspect of Jackson's regression was behind us, and that we no longer needed a pediatric neurologist. I think of him often, and I continue to be thankful I was referred to him by our pediatrician.

I am reminded of the words he said to us during our first visit: "If I'm going to run this show, we're going to slow down and address one medication at a time." He was referring to the three seizure meds that had been prescribed for Jackson by the neurologist I had wanted to whack with his textbook. When he said those words, my first thoughts had been: *Finally, I've found someone to help me with Jackson's neurological needs, and I no longer have to run this show myself.* I had no idea what I was doing and was extraordinarily grateful someone so qualified was taking over.

****

Bill and I celebrated Jackson's success and our hard work by trying, once again, to take the weekend to ourselves that had ended so miserably three years earlier, with Jackson's first seizures. This time, Jennifer agreed to keep the children, and we went only about two hours away by car. Jennifer knew all Jackson's medication and supplements, and we knew we could get home quickly if we had to. We hadn't been alone in three years, and we were so looking forward to the trip.

We decided to go back to the same beach where Bill had asked me to marry him. We had visions of exercising, eating in our favorite restaurants, fitting in a spa treatment, and being intimate without being interrupted. It would be a spectacular weekend.

Other couples with special-needs children have implemented strategies that allow them to maintain their relationships despite exceptional time demands. For example, Laura Marshak and Fran Pollock Prezant write in *Married with Special-Needs Children: A Couples' Guide to Keeping Connected*:

> Emailing each other throughout the day; making a commitment to have at least one conversation every day about their day (not just

their children's day); or taking time off work when the children are at school to be together. In addition, they've found ways to protect and nourish their relationship to include: planning the occasional romantic time for just the two of you; or finding times to prioritize the marriage above all else (relationships with your parents, children, and your career). Healthy marriages do not need to conform to the proportions of this model, but couples with successful marriages do strike a good balance between shared and autonomous space, and an awareness of the marriage itself.[2]

We left for the beach on a Friday morning and would return on Sunday afternoon. This way, we went only one full day without seeing the children, and Jennifer could call us anytime on our cell phones if Jackson or Abby wanted to talk to us. We arrived at lunchtime, went to one of the restaurants we had frequented when we were dating, and had a wonderful meal with a glass of wine. Everything was just as we'd planned. We checked into the hotel and decided to take a nap. That nap set the tone for the rest of our weekend.

I don't think we woke up long enough to do anything but have our next meal and go back to sleep. I'm sure we bathed in there somewhere, but mostly we slept, and slept, and slept some more. Every once in a while, we'd open our eyes, make some utterance toward each other, and drift back into a state of unconsciousness.

Jan Frazier explains this feeling, in *When Fear Falls Away*: "It was like the exhaustion a person feels after the relenting of great pain. It isn't until the pain finally melts from the body that the mind comes to understand what effort the poor body has been expending, just to hold itself together. For it is not only painful to be in pain; it is tiring."[3]

Sunday afternoon arrived before we knew it, and we were on our way home. It was not the weekend we were anticipating, but it was obviously the weekend we needed.

****

In April, we repeated the comprehensive organic profile test on Jackson to see where he was biochemically. We were ecstatic with the results. For the first time since he got sick, Jackson showed no elevated yeast, clostridia, or any other bacteria. The flora in his intestine was finally back in balance. Within two months, we were able to successfully stop the seizure meds; we had achieved another milestone in Jackson's recovery.

On the downside, the test results also showed that Jackson continued to be biochemically imbalanced. Specifically, he still needed more L-carnitine and CoQ10, vitamin B2, folic acid, vitamins C and E, glutathione, and lipoic acid.

My question was this: if Jackson's gut flora was back in balance, then why did he still need all these supplements? The answer: the gut flora being in balance didn't mean his intestine had healed enough to be able to absorb all the nutrients he needed from food, so he continued to be biochemically imbalanced.

Back to the nutritionist we went for another tune-up. Dana increased the levels of CoQ10 and L-carnitine in Jackson's compounded supplement and added vitamins A, E, and C, along with lipoic acid, selenium, and chromium.

The complexity of what the body needs to function normally is amazing. Again, with the enhanced supplements, we saw marked improvement in Jackson's development, especially with his ability to engage with his peers, pay attention and participate in school, and recall language.

I had started working a compressed work schedule, so I could have every other Friday off. I didn't always get them, but when I did, I liked to volunteer in both children's classrooms. Mostly, I wanted to see how they were doing in comparison to their peers. Helping the teachers was secondary but important as well. One Friday, Jackson's teacher asked me to complete a reading exercise with the children. I sat with each child as they read to me. I realized she had given me this task on purpose, so I could see how well Jackson was reading in school.

Some of the children were struggling, and some of them were quite advanced. I was holding cards with sentences on them while the children read them aloud to me. One little girl reached over, took the cards out of my hand, and read like she was capable of charging through *War and Peace*. Other children couldn't make out the words and repeated the same word over several times. Jackson was in the middle of the group, fluid in his reading and right where he was supposed to be. I was thrilled, and the teacher knew it.

Later that same afternoon, I was reading Dr. Seuss's *Horton Hears a Who* to the entire kindergarten class. Being the end of the week, the children were tired, and most were sprawled on the floor. Just as Vlad Vladikoff was about to boil Horton's speck in beezlenut oil, I looked up from the book to see if anyone was paying attention. I found that about two-thirds of the little boys were lying down with their hands down their pants, comforting themselves. But Jackson was not one of them. He was paying attention, and I couldn't wait to go home and tell Bill. Were we passing yet another milestone?

After three and a half years of the acute stage of this illness, I had a very hard time believing that he could ever again be the bright-eyed, curious child who had developed so beautifully until twenty-nine months. However, Jackson's recovery was moving so fast at this point that I was finally beginning to believe that he might fully recover. Regardless, we remained vigilant in dispensing every supplement, keeping every doctor's appointment, and monitoring every developmental milestone.

I think any parent in our situation would tell you that it's easy to put a child like Jackson under a microscope. Every behavior gets questioned as to whether it's typical or a result of a medical or learning difference. I know some of his behavior was typical of a six-year-old little boy, but I was never a six-year-old little boy, and occasionally, his behavior still seemed odd to me.

That spring, when Jackson was still in kindergarten, we reenrolled him in the county soccer program. He wanted to play with his classmates, and to help ensure Jackson would be supported, Bill volunteered to be the assistant coach. It was a completely different experience than it had been just two years earlier. Jackson loved playing with the boys and running up and down the field, and he was proud that his dad was the coach. However, he never quite engaged in the game.

Jackson didn't like to overheat, and he didn't like other children slamming into him—and with all the activity on the field, he quickly lost focus. It was much easier for Jackson to work one-on-one or in a small group than it was to negotiate chaos. To compensate, he ran alongside the other kids, but he didn't really participate in the game. What was encouraging was that he looked forward to practices and wanted to be part of the team.

Many parents have preconceived ideas based on their own childhood experiences of what their children will enjoy. Bill and I both participated in team sports when we were young and wanted Jackson to have some of the same experiences that had helped shape our lives, but we had to adjust our expectations.

The end of the school year came. Jackson was reading on level and was fully proficient in science. His math scores were good, and he was improving in personal and social development. He still didn't have a lot of friends and wasn't invited to many birthday parties, but he was a good friend to those he did have. I was hopeful that additional social skills would come with time. Most of Jackson's issues with friends revolved around his ability to process language and engage. His teacher recommended that Jackson move on to first grade.

The annual review in preparation for first grade went flawlessly. Everyone working with Jackson was supportive of him, recognized his strengths and the areas in which he was delayed, and suggested instructional strategies that would help him catch up. As he had such a successful kindergarten year, his teachers recommended that he receive the same level of support for first grade.

Jennifer again worked with the school's speech pathologist to expand Jackson's goals in receptive and expressive language, and Christine worked with the school's occupational therapist on how to improve Jackson's fine motor and writing capabilities. Earlier in the year, I had a discussion with the special educator who was working with Jackson on recommendations regarding summer programs. She recommended a church-run, private camp for children in preschool through twelfth grade. I was pleasantly surprised to find the camp to be one of the more financially reasonable in the county.

Jackson and I met with the kindergarten and first-grade camp director prior to the first session. She agreed to let Jennifer see Jackson at camp twice a week, with a goal of working on functional language in a setting with other children. They also had a camp nurse, who would give Jackson his digestive enzyme with lunch. The camp day was from nine in the morning until four in the afternoon, and the kids spent a lot of time outside.

Among many things, I worried about how Jackson would handle the heat and if anyone would remind him to drink from his water bottle. My concerns were unfounded; he was very well supported and cared for. In fact, he was finally in an environment that was about having fun and not specifically about his development. He flew down ziplines and went to the pool twice a week. The camp had go-carts, and Jackson was disappointed that he could only ride with his counselor and not yet drive one.

The camp had theme days, with moon bounces and water slides, arts and crafts, and music. At the pond on the property, the kids watched tadpoles turn into frogs and went paddle boating. Jackson loved every minute of it, and I could always tell how much fun he had had based on how filthy he was at the end of the day.

CHAPTER 11

ATTENTION DEFICIT HYPERACTIVITY DISORDER (ADHD)

• • • • • • • • • • • •

Jackson was continuing to make progress, although he had difficulty staying on task in school and at home. I had to believe that as his medical condition continued to resolve, so would his cognitive abilities. To quote Dr. Roberts, "We're going to continue to believe that Jackson will recover fully until he tells us otherwise." Even today, I consistently repeat this quote in my mind. The new school year would come with a series of language, cognitive, and biochemical testing. I felt as if Jackson was under a microscope, but if it would give us the information we needed to help him further recover and reach his fullest potential, then it would be worth it.

Abby was starting kindergarten with the teacher Jackson had the year before. She was a great teacher, and I knew Abby would thrive in her classroom. I watched Abby get on the bus with Jackson on the first day of school. They sat together, and both waved to Bill and me as the bus pulled away. As I had the year before, I arrived at the school before the bus and watched as they both got off and walked into the school building. I got home from work that day in time to meet the afternoon bus and hear all about the first day of kindergarten and first grade.

Jackson was developing and regaining social skills but at a slower pace than that of his academic achievements. In September, one of Bill's nieces got married, and Abby was a flower girl in the wedding. Jackson tried to steal the first dance with the bride; he loved music, and he had turned into quite a dancer. I'm not really sure where he got his moves, but they were spectacular. He wasn't getting them from me, and I can guarantee he didn't get them from his father; Bill would rather eat dirt than dance, and it takes multiple shots of courage to get him on a dance floor. As Jackson and I watched television together, I later realized he had been learning dance steps from TV and movies.

Jackson was becoming friends with a couple of little boys in his class who were as gentle as he was, and the playdates started to come. It was a year of pirates, superheroes, and action figures. I thought he might like to watch *Spiderman* one night, so I put it on, thinking it was the children's version of the movie, and walked away to join Bill. When he checked on Jackson a few minutes later, he found that I had sat our seven-year-old in front of the R-rated version. A particularly violent scene was taking place as Bill walked into the room. He quickly grabbed the remote control and turned the movie off as Jackson flew up the stairs to find me.

Jackson's heart was pounding, and he'd lost the color in his face. It took him about thirty minutes to calm down while sitting in my lap. I might as well have shown him *Alien*. It would be several years before we could get him to watch an action movie he'd never seen before. Regardless, he wanted to be Spiderman that Halloween; apparently, I hadn't traumatized him to the point that he couldn't separate his play from the horror movie.

While Jackson's social skills were improving, I became increasingly frustrated throughout the year with his first-grade teacher's lack of communication. She rarely returned emails if I had a question, nor did she impart much information in face-to-face conversation. Although she was the instructor who spent the majority of time with Jackson during the school day, most of my feedback came from the special educator working with him.

I finally turned inward and told myself to focus on the big picture: Jackson enjoyed going to school every day, he was working at or above level in every subject, and he had good support. Why should his teacher feel the need to stay in close contact with me? My fear of Jackson slipping backward kept me returning like a moth to a flame in monitoring his support systems. But as I had told myself at the beginning of the year, it was time to back away.

That was much easier said than done. I found there was no special formula or approach to being more hands-off. As a parent, you have to know your child and what is right for that child, and I suspect every family's situation is different. However, I did watch intently from afar.

By the end of the first marking period, Jackson had all satisfactory scores—which was great news for us. I don't expect either of my children to be at the top of every class. I want them to always do their best but also to have fun and enjoy life. Living in an area of overachievers, I watch too many children get pushed to their limits and beyond, resulting in a generation of stressed and depressed children. I think children have the cognitive ability to handle a large workload, but they don't have the emotional maturity to handle the pressure, and from my perspective, they shouldn't have to. Especially not a child who was working as hard as Jackson to recover physically, socially, and cognitively.

Although Jackson was at his grade level academically, he wasn't excelling in any subject, with the exception of math computation. He was keeping up in the middle of the pack, which was fantastic for a child with Jackson's history. The areas in which he needed help continued to be completing tasks independently, engaging on his own, meeting goals, following directions, and exercising self-control.

Most of Jackson's limitations in learning skills seemed to be related to an attention deficit. I'm still not sure what his teacher meant by "exercising self-control," as he typically didn't demonstrate impulsive behavior, kept his hands to himself, didn't bother other children, and wasn't disruptive in class. A more communicative teacher might have expanded upon this comment for me.

I got a call from a playground supervisor one afternoon to tell me that another child had told her that Jackson pulled his pants down on the playground that day. I asked her if she could give me any context, as I found it hard to believe Jackson would disrobe on the playground for no reason. She told me that no adult had seen the incident but that she was going to enter the incident in Jackson's permanent record. I strongly suggested that nothing would go in Jackson's permanent record that had not been observed by an adult and assured her I would talk to Jackson when I got home that night.

Jackson had become friendly with a little girl who had also been in his kindergarten class; we'll call her Jane. They had developed a bit of a crush on each other. Suffice it to say that Jane was not the positive influence I would have chosen for Jackson and certainly not one for someone with his still-developing social skills. It turned out Jane had suggested that Jackson might like to "kiss her butt," and apparently Jackson politely offered her his.

Bill and I concluded that Jackson had mooned his first crush; perhaps this was his teacher's definition of "inability to exercise self-control." I called the school the next day and talked to the principal. We all ended up getting a good laugh out of it. But I made it clear to Jackson that he was never to do it again under any circumstances. Jane was also taken to task, and that was the beginning of the end of the first-grade romance.

****

Given Jackson's difficulties in staying on task, we knew the time was approaching when we would need to have him assessed for ADHD. The neurologist had suggested it when we took Jackson off seizure meds, but I had wanted to wait until his intestine was healed and there were no longer any toxins affecting his behavior. I didn't want him to be misdiagnosed in any way or have a diagnosis confused based on too many variables.

He had been tested again for elevated heavy metals by Dana Laake, just before the school year started. The tests showed that he was slightly high in mercury and lead, which can, among other things, lead to inattentiveness and learning disorders. Dr. Roberts explained to me that he probably wasn't absorbing any more mercury or lead in his body than you or me, but being biochemically imbalanced, he wasn't able to clear waste as effectively as someone with a healthy system. One of the most common problems in those with autism is the reduced ability to rid naturally occurring and manufactured toxins. Jackson was taking supplements to support the enzymes and systems responsible for toxin removal.

Jackson still had a hard time settling himself if he was overstimulated. He was being particularly silly one evening— irritatingly obnoxious really—and I asked him why he was behaving that way. Without hesitation, he told me that his "brain felt tied in knots." The neurologist had recommended a neuropsychologist to evaluate Jackson when we were ready.

About a year after the discussion with the neurologist and after Jennifer performed a comprehensive speech and language evaluation, Bill and I agreed that it was time to move forward with the neuropsychology assessment. Jackson was 7.3 years old when Jennifer conducted the testing, and all three components of the test showed he was considered to be within normal limits for his same-age peers, though slightly below his 7.3 years.

In addition, an expressive (the ability to communicate through language) and receptive (the ability to understand what is being said) vocabulary test was conducted. Although Jackson scored an age equivalency of 8.9 in expressive vocabulary, he scored an age equivalency for receptive vocabulary at 6.0 and 6.8. Jennifer thought that the lower scores may have been associated with attention and focus on that particular day, but a movement break did not seem to affect his ability to focus on the test.

Jennifer performed a last test called a Comprehensive Assessment of Spoken Language (CASL), which included testing on sixteen factors, such as antonyms, synonyms, sentence completion, and paragraph comprehension. Jackson scored anywhere from 5.0 years to 7.8 across the sixteen factors, with the majority of scores falling in the 6.5- to 7-year range. These scores may sound grim to some parents, but they were great news for us: Jackson had caught up to the point where his language processing, on average, was about only six months behind his typical peers.

The recommendations coming from Jennifer's ensuing report were that Jackson should...

> undergo neuropsychological testing to investigate his attention, focus, and processing abilities as his ability to attend and focus is

variable. He should be evaluated for sensory integration issues by an occupational therapist, and he should continue to be seen for private speech-language therapy to focus on non-literal language skills, inferencing, and problem solving. The issue of word finding should also be further investigated.

I had no clue what neuropsychology was. Again, I turned to the internet. According to the National Academy of Neuropsychology:

> Neuropsychology is a branch of clinical psychology that studies how the brain and nervous system affect how we function on a daily basis. Unlike the use of neuroimaging techniques such as MRI, CT scans and EEG where the focus is on the nervous system structures, neuropsychology seeks to understand how the various components of the brain are able to do their jobs.
>
> Clinical neuropsychology makes use of various assessment methods to ascertain function and dysfunction and applies this knowledge to evaluate, treat and rehabilitate individuals with suspected or demonstrated neurological or psychological problems.[1]

I was slightly nervous about this evaluation, as I still had the smallest of doubts about whether or not a neuropsychology evaluation might tell us that Jackson had high-functioning autism or Asperger's syndrome. Why would this diagnosis bother me, given everything we had been through and all the progress Jackson had made? Because such a diagnosis would tell us that despite the remarkable progress he was making and all the intensive work we had accomplished together, he would surely face additional challenges as he matured. Rational or not, this was one more admission of my fears for my child. As Lorna Bradley says in *Special Needs Parenting: From Coping to Thriving*:

> As parents of children with special needs, it is a constant battle to advocate for a child in a culture that pushes them to the margins, defining them as "less than" simply because they are "different than." The differences in our children are often seen as 'tragic' by others—and unfairly so ... [2]
>
> All parents have an image of a child that they hope to have one day. That image is filled with hopes and dreams and expectations. There is an expected order to life with developmental milestones leading toward maturity and independence. It is not so much having an expectation of perfection in the child, but rather an image of how that child's life is expected to unfold.[3]

It's appropriate and normal to grieve, and parents with children with differences grieve over and over again, with each missed milestone. Bill and I were no exception. I wasn't grieving for myself but for abilities that Jackson was struggling to learn and or regain. We both want Jackson and Abby to ultimately leave the nest and experience independence and lives of their own when the time is appropriate. According to Lorna Bradley:

> The grief felt by parents of children with special needs is unique in a few ways. First, it is often accompanied by guilt.
>
> Second, it is chronic in nature, raising its head again and again, why is guilt attached to grieving for a child? If grieving for a person who has died, or for a lost job, or for the lost companionship of a friend who moved away, people expect to feel that grief. They don't typically feel guilty for grieving those losses because grief would be expected in those situations.
>
> Grieving for a child who lives and remains with you daily is an unexpected grief and it goes hand-in-hand with guilt. One parent shared with me the guilt she felt for grieving for her daughter's Down syndrome ... simply by experiencing and acknowledging grief, she felt she was saying that her child was not good enough.[4]

On the other hand, what if the neuropsychologist's findings were yet another confirmation that Jackson was not autistic, and my hypothesis was still valid—that too many children are being put on the autism spectrum? These children who have very different issues and needs could potentially recover. I Googled the neuropsychologist, read his website, was pleased with the depth of his practice, and called for an appointment.

****

Meanwhile, I learned what a neuropsychological evaluation entails. At the time, according to the practice of the Stixrud Group:

> The Neuropsychological Evaluation takes approximately eight hours (conducted in one or two session, depending on age and stamina) and includes the following testing categories:
>
> - Intellectual abilities testing.
> - Educational achievement testing.
> - Neuropsychological test battery: Testing in the areas of attentional functioning, organizational skills, motor skills, sensory-perceptual functioning, receptive and expressive language abilities, visual-perceptual and visuo-constructive abilities, reasoning and problem-solving abilities, learning and memory.
> - Personality screening to assess personality style, current coping skills, emotional state, and well-being. [5]

Based on Jackson's history and the progress he had made to date, the neuropsychologist oversaw the evaluation himself. We worked collaboratively with him and his associate over the next several weeks to complete the testing and document the results. I took Jackson for two visits, where we spent most of the day; he was allowed short play breaks and a break for lunch. As usual, Jackson's personality won over the psychologists, and they were able to get as much cooperation out of him as possible. Testing like this would require extensive dedication from any child, and much more so from one with Jackson's history.

Bill and I still weren't clear on the residual effects that encephalopathy, toxicity, and seizures might be having on Jackson's cognitive, physical, and social development. It was obvious he had an attention deficit, but what other results of his earlier illness might he struggle with? He might have had ADHD even if he hadn't gotten so sick when he was twenty-nine months. I was banking on this testing telling me the answers to these questions. But ultimately, only time and development would provide the answers we were looking for.

During the second visit, I was sitting in the waiting room wondering what the doctors might find, when the associate brought Jackson out for a break.

I asked her how it was going, and she immediately said, "He has a hard time focusing."

"I know," I replied. "That's why we're here."

She looked at me again. "He has a *really* hard time focusing." Sadly, I knew that too.

After several weeks, we sat down with both psychologists to receive their assessment and recommendations for school and other aspects of growth and development. Bill and I invited Jennifer to attend the meeting with us. We hoped she could help us interpret anything we didn't understand from the assessment and help us implement any new strategies recommended with regard to language processing.

The neuropsychological report told us the following:

> Jackson presented as a sweet and charming boy who separated easily from his mother. His social interactions were generally appropriate for his age.

> However, it was noted that his eye contact during testing was variable, that he had some

difficulty with social reciprocity, and that he would interrupt the examiner or continue to talk even after a conversation had ended. It was also noted that Jackson had significant difficulty sustaining his attention, even within this highly structured one-to-one testing session.

From the start, he was very self-directed and required several prompts to return his attention to tasks. He had particular difficulty sustaining his attention during verbally-based tasks and made frequent off-task comments or interrupted the examiner to ask a question. He was not consistently motivated by stickers and requested frequent "stand-up" and play breaks ...

Some staring spells were observed during the evaluation, which appeared to be lapses in attention, rather than seizure activity ... Jackson's speech was normal in rate and rhythm, but he sometimes spoke softly and ... had difficulty organizing his ideas. Jackson's mood and attitude toward testing were generally appropriate ...

Overall, Jackson was cooperative with the examiner and appeared to put forth his best effort; however, his inattention and heightened activity interfered with his performance on several tasks. Therefore, the results of testing might slightly underestimate his true abilities in some areas.

The assessment indicated that Jackson's verbal strengths and weaknesses were consistent with the testing Jennifer had performed:

> Jackson had significant difficulty sustaining his attention within this highly structured testing environment; he was easily distracted by outside noises as well as his own internal thoughts ... Jackson also exhibited marked weaknesses in executive functioning, which refers to the mental organizational processes associated with initiating, implementing, monitoring, and revising strategies and plans of action.

All was consistent with textbook definitions of ADHD. In addition, the report indicated that Jackson was "below average in information processing and writing output speed, which affects his ability to work efficiently under timed conditions."

Bill and I found the diagnostic impressions documented in the report to be somewhat discouraging. The report continued:

> While adults may be able to give Jackson feedback and guide him along socially, his peers are more likely to become frustrated with him, which poses risks for later social difficulties and poor self-esteem.

> Fortunately, Jackson is a very sweet boy with a sunny disposition who is a joy to be around. He has been through a tremendous amount of stress for someone his age, and even his neuropsychological profile, which reflects many entirely age-appropriate abilities, cannot

capture the amazing strength of this boy or the remarkable resilience that he has shown following a very frightening period of time for him and for his family. The abilities he currently has are a testament to his hard work and the support of his family, who were persistent in getting him the services that he needs.

A diagnosis of ADHD was documented—predominantly inattentive type; a mixed receptive expressive language disorder; cognitive disorder (not otherwise specified) in processing speed; and learning disorder (not otherwise specified) in math fluency and writing output speed and production.

The psychologists agreed that Jackson's academic placement was appropriate at the time and recommended that, as first grade came to an end, his current level of support in the classroom continue for second grade. They also suggested that he might need additional support as he transitioned from second to third grade, as academics progress from "learning to read" to "reading to learn," and work becomes more complex.

The neuropsychologists recommended classroom accommodations, such as preferential seating close to teachers and away from distractions, and extended time to complete tasks such as testing or timed activities. Suggestions around general teaching included helping Jackson manage his workload by breaking larger tasks into smaller, more manageable components, avoiding overload, and introducing new information in a familiar context.

The report also included specific suggestions addressing academic strategies, including reading fluency and comprehension, writing, and math; the use of an executive tutor (who would help him plan and organize his work and other tasks); relaxation techniques such as yoga, to help him focus and resist distractions in the environment; and improved physical fitness to provide the motivation and confidence to learn new skills.

****

It was also at this time that the neuropsychologists suggested a medication consultation about the possibility of starting Jackson on a stimulant medication for ADHD. This would help regulate his attention and ability to stay on task and potentially help Jackson maintain self-esteem through participation in outside activities that he enjoyed and at which he could excel.

Having heard all this from a professional, I was energized, all over again, to make additional changes to our routine and therapies in providing Jackson with the resources he needed to grow in every dimension. However, children have a mind of their own. Jackson didn't want to take yoga. He already worked with teachers and para-educators in his classroom, speech pathologists, occupational therapists, and three different doctors; he didn't want any more.

Jackson's reality was that he wanted to be a kid and play; all these recommendations were seemingly extra work that would put more demands on him. My reality was that all these suggestions, again, came with an extensive time commitment and a price tag. We were still paying for full-time child care, speech, and OT, and now I needed to find an executive coach to tutor him. I did hire an academic tutor to work with him at home to ensure he understood concepts and got his work completed and turned in on time. He eventually did get that executive coach but years later, when his work in high school became much more complex.

I sent a copy of the neuropsychologist's report to Dr. Roberts, delivered a copy to Jackson's teachers, and put one in his permanent school record. Dr. Roberts and I also spoke about the pros and cons of medicating children for ADHD. Among many things, she explained to me that not all ADHD medications work for each child, and finding the right medication can require a process. She suggested that before we did anything, we would need to consult again with the neurologist to discuss the recommended stimulant medication for ADHD, because some ADHD medications are contraindicated in children who have had seizures.

I also talked to our pediatrician, who was encouraged by the progress Jackson was making and with the outcome of the evaluation. He indicated to me that if Jackson came through everything he'd been through with "a little ADHD, we'll take it and be happy." I couldn't have agreed more; albeit challenging at times, at least ADHD is something identifiable and treatable.

Although he was a wonderful human being, I had hoped we'd never have to see the neurologist for a professional visit again. But back we went to the pediatric epilepsy clinic. I told the doctor about the comment Jackson had made indicating his "brain felt tied in knots." This led to an extremely productive discussion about the pros and cons of medicating children for attention deficit hyperactivity disorder. Most ADHD medications are basically stimulants, and I had read that many people can become addicted to the medication, as it increases brain function and processing abilities.

The words the neurologist imparted were invaluable. His experience showed that some children who are not medicated grow up to self-medicate with alcohol and drugs, in an attempt to overcome their day-to-day difficulties. From the school nurse, I heard another message: she said it's not necessarily the children who abuse their ADHD meds but more likely some of the parents who help themselves to their children's medication. I find that incredibly sad, for many reasons.

The neurologist gave me a list of medications that would be relatively safe for Jackson to take. I took the list to Dr. Roberts. The one that she favored was among those the neurologist had preferred; the pediatrician agreed as well. As with the seizure meds, we had to titrate the ADHD drug, so as not to give Jackson too much.

Because the drugs are amphetamines, they can commonly cause jitters, anxiety, high blood pressure, and increased heart rate. Although I understand these side effects are typically mild, there seems to be a fine line between a therapeutic dose and too much. We left Jackson on the lowest dose for about a week, knowing that we would not see a therapeutic result. I kept in very close contact with his teachers that week, monitoring for adverse effects.

The next week, we went to what I thought was the highest dose we could give him and were disappointed when we again saw no therapeutic effect. I wondered how many meds we'd have to go through before we found one that would work for Jackson. I called Dr. Roberts to suggest we needed to try a different drug but was encouraged to find Jackson could take a higher dose of the same medication. As always, I introduced medications or increased dosages on a weekend, so I could observe firsthand any changes in behavior. I knew Jackson's teachers would be pleased with what they saw the third week.

It was mid-May when we started the medication. Our goal was to have Jackson on a therapeutic dose before the end of the school year, so we could see how he would perform academically.

The response was extraordinary. That Monday, his teachers each sent me an email. Jackson was a different child, they wrote; he was engaged, participative, and talkative. I never found Jackson to be an uncooperative child, except at his sickest, when he was miserable. But on the medication, he could follow directions more easily and do what was asked of him after only one or two requests. Also encouraging was that not only did the medication help with Jackson's attention deficit and executive functioning, it increased his processing speed and allowed him to recall information and access his language much more easily.

I was ecstatic that the first medication we tried was working. Despite my enthusiasm, there are side effects of ADHD medications we needed to watch for, such as decreased appetite, mild headache or stomachache, and weight loss or suppressed height growth rate. These symptoms typically resolve when the medication is stopped. To try to compensate for diminished growth rate, we timed Jackson's medication so he would eat as much as possible.

Knowing Jackson wouldn't eat much of his lunch, we gave him a big breakfast with lots of protein before medicating him for the school day. One positive aspect of most ADHD medications is that they wear off after the prescribed dose and don't stay or build up in your system. The drug wore off after about seven hours, so he would eat a significant snack when he got home from school and get a good dinner. However, our efforts were in vain; Jackson's growth rate did slow down but continued to track at a consistent pace.

First grade ended on a high note. Jackson had been off of his seizure meds for a year, and we'd seen no sign of any type of seizure. He was medicated for ADHD and showed marked improvement, and many of the satisfactory marks he had earned during the first grading period had moved to outstanding. The same level of support would be continued for second grade, including special education, speech, and occupational therapy.

After volunteering in a few of Jackson's classes, I recognized there were many children with social, behavioral, and academic differences. I wondered how many of them had been put under a microscope like Jackson. Sometimes the distinction between a child with special needs and typical seven-year-old little boy behavior is easy to miss.

For instance, Jackson's teacher that year was very concerned because he "picked his nose." But all I had to do was look around the classroom to observe the majority of children with a finger up a nostril. I told the neuropsychologist about the teacher's concern, and her response to me was, "How ridiculous. They all pick their noses." I guess this was another example of the teacher's definition of "exercising self-control."

We spent a week at the beach shortly after school was out for the summer. This vacation was as different as night and day from previous years, thanks to the ADHD medication. Jackson was focused on the beach and spent much of each day learning to boogie board. He stayed with us and his aunts and uncles on the beach and didn't wander off or want to go do something else. For the first time since the kids were born, Bill and I could actually sit on the beach and read a book—not for very long, but then I don't know anyone with five- and seven-year-old children who can sit for very long to do anything.

That summer, Jackson went back to the camp where he had his first experience swimming in dirty water with snapping turtles and frogs. He came home one night with dirt all over his shirt, including several muddy footprints. I asked him how he got stepped on.

"I didn't get stepped on, Mom," he said. "I took my shirt off and left it by the side of the pond when we went canoeing."

"How did it get so muddy?" I asked.

"Well, my friend and I decided to jump out of the canoe in the middle of the pond."

"How did you get back in your canoe?"

"We didn't," he said. "We swam to shore, and that's when my shirt got stepped on and muddy."

I don't think I ever found out how the canoe got back to shore. I wondered if we would need an antibiotic for some obscure bacteria he had picked up in the pond. But we didn't. I was actually thrilled that my special-needs child with learning differences was jumping out of canoes to swim with snapping turtles. What active, curious, and adventurous child wouldn't love that?

CHAPTER 12

ADVOCATING

· · · · · · · · · · · ·

I was transplanting lilies and irises again, the same lilies and irises I've moved from house to house, the plants that originally came from my mother's garden. Although she's gone, when I'm in my garden, I feel as though she's always with me. Most of my perennials were products of her yard. I've nurtured them every spring, just as she did, mostly because she instilled in me her love of beauty, creativity, and gardening, and partly because I'm afraid that if I let anything happen to them, she'll know I killed her plants.

Jackson, now eight, was just finishing the second grade. Bill had taken Abby, six, to Upstate New York to visit his parents for the Memorial Day weekend, so it was just Jackson and me in the backyard. He was desperately trying to entertain himself, until I gave up my chores to take him to the neighborhood pool that had just opened for the season. Initially, he'd joined me in the garden with enthusiasm, but after bringing me a garbage can for yard trim and picking up the weeds I had pulled, he had sat down in a pile of dirt with a hand shovel to dig for worms.

Worms are much more interesting to an eight-year-old boy than pulling weeds. But the worms wouldn't keep his interest much longer with the promise of water ahead of him. Jackson loved to swim. In fact, he loved to be in any water—the pool, sprinkler, bathtub, shower, even the dirty pond with snapping turtles and frogs.

It had taken me about thirty minutes to get sunscreen on Jackson—some children with sensory integration issues don't like lotion on their bodies because it feels sticky to them. We finally made it to the pool, but the water was too cold for me; the late-spring sun hadn't been shining on it long enough to warm it to an acceptable temperature for anyone other than an enthusiastic child. Jackson went right in. He still didn't tolerate heat well, and the pressure and the coolness of the water against his body restored his energy.

Before I knew it, he had mustered his courage and was standing on the diving board with his goggles on—Jackson didn't like water in his eyes. The lifeguard blew his whistle and told him he had to take his goggles off. I thought the summer season might end for Jackson on the first day the pool opened and that he might just ask to go home. He didn't, but he retreated from the diving board back to the shallow end of the pool, where he could live by his own rules, at least temporarily.

The next weekend, Jackson watched Abby fly off the diving board with reckless abandon and couldn't stay away any longer, with or without goggles. The first jump turned into several, and he no longer seemed to notice the water in his eyes. He had passed another milestone. At that point, I found that Jackson conquered most rites of childhood about six months to a year behind his peers.

In addition to swimming, one of Jackson's favorite things to do was play games on the Wii, especially some of the sports. He'd taken a particular liking to golf and wanted me to take him to play nine holes that same weekend. I explained to him that playing the real game wasn't like playing Wii and that maybe we should try the driving range first. He'd gotten three golf clubs for Christmas, so off we went with his driver, putter, and seven iron and my 1950s Tommy Armor clubs that I had inherited from my father. We each got a bucket of balls, and then I gave him one quick lesson. I showed him how to tee up his ball and stood back and watched him smack it about a hundred yards.

I stood at the tee behind him, taking one pathetic swing after another, while he consistently hit straight for about fifty yards. When we each finished our buckets, he wanted to go practice putting, and then he insisted on one more bucket of balls at the driving range. I started to resist, as my hand was already looking rather raw, but I gave in to his pleading. We split the bucket; he had a great time, and I walked away with a bleeding blister. Jackson showed so much enthusiasm for these types of activities. He felt better and didn't tire as quickly as before.

****

Eight months earlier, at the beginning of Jackson's second-grade school year, I had gone to meet with his new teachers to explain his history. I hoped to convince them that my child deserved their support. It was a ritual visit I had done every school year. As usual, I accomplished my goal of reciting Jackson's history. But this year, I walked away feeling as though all the teachers thought I was an overprotective mother who couldn't let her fledgling spread his wings and leave the nest. They looked at how well he was doing at that point. They didn't have the context; they hadn't lived through the history we had. They probably wondered why I continued to advocate for him.

Near the end of first grade, the neuropsychologist had given Jackson a diagnosis of ADHD with an expressive and receptive language-processing disorder. From what I have learned, ADHD comes in three forms: inattentive type, hyperactive-impulsive type, and combined type. Jackson's diagnosis was primarily inattentive type; he does not show typical signs of hyperactivity. After years of working with neurologists, developmental pediatricians, and speech pathologists, we knew all this. But to continue to get services through the school system, we had to have it formally documented.

Since annual reviews are done at the end of each school year, and Jackson had started on ADHD medication at the end of first grade, I asked for a review ninety days into second grade. A ninety-day review gives a parent the opportunity to see if the IEP is being implemented appropriately. IEP meetings are generally scheduled as a one-hour meeting that typically lasts for about three to four. The purpose is to discuss your special child's needs and determine what, if any, support they need to learn the curriculum for the school year. During the meeting, you sit around a conference table with multiple school administrators in the county who know nothing about your child—and the principal, teachers, and therapists who truly have your child's best interests at heart.

In contrast to IEP meetings, a typical parent-child conference lasts about fifteen to twenty minutes and involves only the child's teacher and the parents. It's a much easier process.

IEP meetings can go two ways. You can have an amazing experience, where you feel as though everyone who interacts with your child in any way would do anything to help him or her learn and grow to their fullest potential. Or you can come out of an IEP meeting intellectually and emotionally exhausted. School systems have to work within their budgets, but if more money were allocated for special programs, our children would consistently get the support they need. Parents wouldn't have to fight an uphill battle every year when advocating for their child.

At this particular meeting, I found that the acting principal was an intern. The speech pathologist and occupational therapists were new to the school. The special educator was new to the county—and had decided after one week of knowing Jackson that it would be a good idea to cut his services. In addition, one of the school administrators wanted to change his diagnosis, in an attempt to support cutting his services.

I asked the administrator, "Have you ever met Jackson?"

"No."

"Are you a neurologist?" I asked.

"No."

"A developmental pediatrician? A neuropsychologist?"

"No."

"Then what qualifies you to change my son's medical diagnosis?" I vehemently asked. She was silent.

I turned my next question to the room. "Have any of you read Jackson's recent IEP or neuropsychology report?"

The answer from all was "No."

This is why I continued to advocate for Jackson. I never took my eyes off all the multiple variables that had to come together to ensure his ongoing recovery and allow him to reach his full potential.

In my most controlled and professional voice, yet with chin quivering and tears welling up in my eyes, I told everyone around the table that they clearly weren't taking my child's educational needs seriously.

Bill interjected and told me to stop it. At the same time, Suzie announced, "Jackson had been autistic, and he deserves better attention than he seems to be getting."

It was about this time that my rage got the best of me, not because of Suzie's comment (Jackson was never diagnosed with autism) but because of the lack of attention and respect with which these educational *professionals* seemed to be treating my child. They didn't appear to be focusing on Jackson's individual needs.

I ended the meeting and requested a much smaller meeting in one week, with the principal and the special educator alone. I have to admit that we've only had one or two other IEP meetings as bad as this one. Deep breathing works momentarily, but full recovery from these types of IEP meetings can take me about a week.

In the interim, I met with Jackson's classroom teacher to ask her opinion on how he was doing in the classroom. Since classroom teachers spend the most time with the students, they tend to know your child better than any others in the school system. Most who worked with Jackson loved his sweet nature and great sense of humor and admired the amazing progress he had made to this point. As I expected, his teacher was honest with me and didn't think it would be to Jackson's advantage to cut his services.

I met with the principal and the special educator, or resource teacher, as they're called, the next week. The resource teacher wanted to do less "pull out" of the classroom with Jackson and have him do more work with his peers. I was all for that, as long as he was grasping foundational concepts and got enough support in the classroom to keep him on task. We also discussed instructional strategies that might motivate him, things like checklists and reward systems. As a result of the meeting, a para-educator was moved into the classroom to work with him and a handful of other children, the IEP was implemented, and those who had not read his neuropsychology report did so and got to know him better.

Jackson's report card came at the end of the first marking period with six subjects marked as outstanding—including speaking—four areas of math, and science. All other subjects were marked as satisfactory, with no "needs improvement." The report card indicated that most of his learning skills were completed independently but that he still needed frequent prompting to complete his class work, engage in tasks on his own, and follow oral and written directions. Given where we'd been with him, this was good.

With as much speech therapy as Jackson had, I would have been surprised if he hadn't gotten an outstanding in speaking. He still attended private speech once a week to help overcome the language-processing problem, and he was receiving an hour a week of speech in school. He was always very articulate except at his sickest, but he couldn't consistently access his language. He no longer needed private occupational therapy at this time, but he was still getting help in school to overcome some writing challenges, mostly due to muscle weakness in his hands.

In early December, we had a follow-up appointment with the nutritionist who was helping us with some of Jackson's supplements. As Jackson continued to be biochemically imbalanced, Dr. Roberts wanted him to have a tune-up about every six months, which typically involved testing blood and urine. As Jackson had grown, he'd been able to do without some of his medication and supplements, but we had to increase others. He was still taking a mineral and a vitamin B supplement compound to meet his specific needs, a digestive enzyme, probiotics, natural and synthetic antihistamines, glutathione, an omega-3 fatty acid, and vitamin D.

****

Christmas in the second grade was all about Legos. Jackson could take any Lego construction toy for almost any age group and put it together with unbelievable focus and precision. He received several Lego sets intended for fourteen-year-olds. We watched him sit intently and build for hours. He also loved to build with K'nex construction sets, which he approached with the same determination. We have learned that children with ADHD can actually hyper focus when particularly interested in a subject or task, and Jackson is no exception. He may need frequent prompting to stay on some tasks at school and at home, but you sometimes can't distract him from an undertaking if he's enjoying it and is fully engaged.

Jackson loves to see how things operate. Like his father, a civil and environmental engineer, Jackson is much more interested in the mechanics of something than in the actual object. We were visiting Bill's parents soon after his eighty-nine-year-old father had gotten a lift chair to make it easier for him to get in and out of his recliner. Abby wanted to ride up and down in the chair and play with the remote control, whereas Jackson wanted to crawl underneath it to see how it worked. Mostly Abby wanted Jackson to ride with her. I suspect that more than mere companionship, she wanted to see whether she could make her brother catapult across the living room by hitting some eject button. Much to her dismay, the chair moved too slowly.

That same winter, we discovered a four-story indoor splash park about three hours from our house, and I thought the kids would love to go for a long weekend. I spoke to a few parents who had taken their children and got mixed reviews. Everyone I talked to said the kids had a great time, but the parents could only stand it for about twenty-four hours. I thought twenty-four hours sounded much more tolerable than one of those party places where on a Saturday or Sunday afternoon there are about fifty birthdays going on at any one time. I can stand those for about five minutes before I feel like I've been deposited directly into hell.

We made reservations and thought we'd be able to check another item off the good-parents list. Much to our surprise,

Bill and I had as much fun as Jackson and Abby. We all must have gone up and down those four stories of stairs a hundred times. Jackson wanted to go on every slide, no matter how steep, fast, twisted, or where it dumped you at the bottom. Abby was almost there with him, but a little more reluctant on a slide called the "Howling Tornado." I was forced to "Howl the Tornado" just once, after which it took me about ten minutes to catch my breath and get my heart rate back to a normal rhythm. But Jackson and Bill went down countless times.

****

Abby had subtle ways of reminding me that she knew that Jackson was special. Not because of his illness and recovery but because, from her perspective, he's been able to do seemingly special things that didn't include her. She had to attend all his speech and OT sessions with our after-school babysitter. She watched him jump in ball pits, play catch, swing on ziplines, run obstacle courses, color, and "play" with Jennifer.

This recognition hit me like a ton of bricks one night when both kids were arguing over who would sit in my lap. We were watching TV, and at six and eight, they were getting big enough that it was no longer comfortable to have both of them in one lap. I suggested that each could sit for five minutes and then trade places.

They didn't like that idea. The fight was on, each trying to push the other off my lap; of course, I was the one who got hit in the chin with an elbow. I lost my patience and sent them both to their rooms. Abby came back about five minutes later, handed me a folded-up piece of paper, and ran back to her room. The note said, "Six-year-old little girls need their mommies too. You don't have to yell at me." It was obvious she felt neglected. But I didn't know if it was just at that moment or in general.

My hunch was that it was in general, and I would need to watch her more closely. Kate Strohm writes in *Being the Other One: Growing Up with a Brother or Sister Who Has Special Needs*:

> Siblings of children with differences can miss out on attention from parents; learn to put the needs of others before their own; at times they may wish they too had special needs; may act out in order to gain attention; may feel pressure to be perfect in order to gain attention and to make things right for their parents; and may feel resentment that the child with special needs is being spoiled, that s/he is being treated differently and being allowed to get away with inappropriate behavior.[1]

I started dreaming up all sorts of special activities I could do alone with Abby. Bill was coaching Jackson's soccer team, so I signed Abby and me up for parent-and-child tennis lessons. I had played when I was younger and thought it might be something I could help her with. I gave her pedicures and painted her toenails pink, which she loved; we watched movies; and she asked to hear stories about me when I was a little girl. We spent a lot of time at paint-your-own pottery, where I created some absolutely hideous things that I stashed in the back of a cabinet. Abby's work, on the other hand, was displayed prominently.

Jackson had fun for the past couple of fall and spring seasons playing soccer. However, it's the kind of sport that takes lots of concentration on the field, and all the action was still difficult for Jackson to process. At one game, I heard some of the other children make comments about his ability, and I knew that soccer wasn't going to last much longer for him. One little boy looked at me one afternoon, not knowing that I was Jackson's mother, and said, "Jackson's a little slow."

At this age, most of the other children were starting to take the game seriously, and Jackson was still out to have fun. He wanted to play and be part of the team, but he seemed to follow alongside the other children, instead of truly being part of the game. The last thing I wanted to do was leave Jackson in a sport where he would be made fun of by other kids; that would run the risk of undermining the confidence he had built.

****

Alternative therapies seemed to come up as necessary throughout our journey with Jackson. I didn't typically seek them with determined purpose but more or less stumbled upon them as I learned about them in my research. Some were introduced to me.

Jackson's speech pathologist introduced me to energy therapy in the spring of 2009. Just as I have with all alternative therapies we've tried with Jackson, I sought to understand it. At the time, the energy practitioner I found described energy therapy in this way:

> The human energy system is a network of interacting, multidimensional energies composing our spiritual, mental, emotional, and physical selves. If these interrelated energies become imbalanced, there may be resulting physical or emotional challenges. An energy medicine practitioner assesses and facilitates the rebalancing of an individual's energy system to promote optimal holistic health.

I realized that I had been going to an energy healer for years. One of the things that prevented me from atrophying as we worked through Jackson's illness was regular massage, and the massage therapist that my internist had recommended was also a Reiki master. Reiki was one form of energy therapy that had helped me stay relaxed—when I took the time to go.

I made an appointment to meet the energy therapist myself, to see what affect her work had on me. After one session, I was hooked, I hadn't felt so relaxed and grounded in years. As we thought it might be helpful in improving Jackson's processing speed, I made an appointment for him, and after about two or three sessions, several weeks apart, both Bill and I noticed a difference in the speed with which he could tell a story.

After a rocky start, the year went well. Jackson asked me during a particularly violent thunderstorm if he could go take a shower—a rare request, I assure you.

"No, water attracts lightning, and you might get zip-zapped," I told him.

He looked at me very seriously and said, "You mean water conducts electricity?"

"Yes," I said. "It does."

"What else conducts electricity?" he asked.

"Go ask your father," I told him. *Zip-zapped? Do I think he's still four?* I asked myself.

****

By the end of the school year, the classroom teacher had taken away Jackson's checklists, as he was able to complete most tasks independently. Jackson's second-grade teacher was very attuned to his needs; she was also proactive in communicating with the other students. Teaching is about meeting our children's needs and helping them learn and grow and not about catering to parents' wants. However, this teacher went the extra mile; I never had to wonder how Jackson was doing or what he needed to be working on at home. She advocated for him in school almost as much as I did.

Not having to wonder what was going on in the classroom made my life much less stressful. He ended the school year with outstanding marks in nine subjects, which included speaking, math, science, two reading scores, listening comprehension, social studies, and music. At this point, he was also exhibiting all learning skills independently and no longer needed frequent prompting in the areas in which he had needed help at the beginning of the year.

With second grade coming to an end, the dreaded annual review was two days away. I had become leery of IEP meetings from our first, when Jackson was three and we met the county school administrators for the first time. I was even more leery after the difficult review ninety days into second grade. The primary school that both children attended only went through the second grade, so Jackson would go to a new school in the fall for third grade.

The annual review to prepare for third grade went as well as any. Two resource teachers from Jackson's new school attended the meeting, to help make the transition to the new environment. In anticipation of meeting the new teachers, I took a copy of Jackson's neuropsychology report to share. One of them immediately picked up on his processing speed and asked if his score was with medication or without. I told her definitely without, and she seemed somewhat relieved.

The occupational therapist who had worked with Jackson throughout second grade had just completed a therapy reevaluation that concluded he no longer needed OT. She opened her comments by putting her hand over her heart and telling us, "First, let me say that I love Jackson. He has a very special place in my heart." Tears were in her eyes, and I knew she saw in him what so many of us do: a smart, loving, empathic child who had courageously endured more in his eight short years than many of us do in a lifetime.

The services he had been receiving were specifically to address fine motor skills, visual motor skills, and written communication. The OT's summary stated:

> Jackson is a second-grade student with an educational disability of Other Health Impairment ... he writes with consistent legibility, appropriate sizing and spacing between words, and age-appropriate speed. Based on a review of Jackson's occupational therapy progress, Jackson's functional level, and Jackson's needs in school, it is recommended that the IEP committee consider discharge from occupational therapy services.

Just one year before, after his neuropsychology evaluation, we had been concerned that his writing speed would hold him back and that he would need to learn to type in third grade to be able to keep up. And now, here we were, ending OT through the school system because he tested at age level! His private OT had come to the same conclusion months earlier, and we had dropped that service as well.

By the end of the year, based on the facts that his teacher was able to reduce his support in the classroom, that he was at grade level in reading and written language (although he still struggled with detail), and that he was at grade level with support in math, we all agreed that the hours of support that Jackson received per week could be reduced from twenty-one to fifteen for the next year. The IEP indicated that Jackson was still below age expectancy for oral language, due to receptive and expressive language skills as well as focus and attention.

One of the new resource teachers asked what kind of classroom would benefit Jackson. I suggested that he would need a teacher who was supportive and kind, yet structured and firm. Jackson remained a perceptive and sensitive child who was fully aware of turmoil or chaos around him. The teachers felt they had the perfect fit for him. Bill and I walked away from the meeting with high hopes for third grade.

We celebrated Jackson's successes that night; he had graduated from private- and school-provided OT, and we could finally reduce the number of hours of support he needed in the classroom. From our perspective, he was doing well academically, and we were impressed with the resource teachers who would be supporting him throughout third grade.

CHAPTER 13

RESILIENCE

· · · · · · · · · · · ·

We found a new vacation spot in August 2009. My friend Liz's
in-laws own a house on a lake in the Adirondack Mountains
and were generous enough to invite us for a week. To be honest,
I'm not sure if they invited us or if we invited ourselves; I
just remember it was a mutually agreeable arrangement. Bill
had gone to college with Liz's husband, and Liz and I had
worked together years before. We'd known the entire family
for some time. We rented a house in the same development as
our friends, and the children were able to run back and forth
between the two houses. The family was more than generous
with their home, hospitality, and boat.

Jackson and Abby learned to fish that summer. As I recall,
Abby caught the first fish and promptly dropped it on the dock.
Bill, Jackson, and Abby were all jumping up and down trying to
catch it as I watched it slip through their fingers and flop around
at their feet. It wasn't much bigger than a robust guppy. Bill's
persistence finally prevailed, and the poor little fish finally made
it back to its natural habitat. It's probably about a foot long now
and likely has never returned to swim anywhere near that dock.

Fishing was fun, but the highlight of the vacation was doing
flips off the dock and tubing behind the boat. As Jackson watched
with some trepidation, we taught him the hand signals for "go
faster," "slow down," and "stop." Despite the depth and breadth
of the lake, he dropped into the water and climbed into the tube.
As we gave the boat some gas, I watched the smile spread across
his face. He immediately gave the signal for "go faster," and he

continued to give the same signal until Abby and the other children started complaining that Jackson's turn had been long enough.

We also did some hiking that vacation to a place called Rocky Mountain. Jackson ran straight up the mountain with the other children, leaving Bill and me in his dust. We were sure we'd find him dangling from a cliff by the time we got to the top. But we found him standing in awe of the spectacular view of the lake from the mountaintop. Just a few years earlier, he wouldn't have felt well enough to make the short walk to the foot of the mountain, much less climb it. After so many years of illness and therapies, it was tremendous to watch both children grow and adapt to the newfound freedom we had as a family. It was such a remarkable week for us that we planned on returning the next year.

We still had to travel with all Jackson's medication, supplements, and gluten-free foods. Most out-of-the-way little towns aren't stocked with any specialty products, so I always made sure that, at least, we had palatable gluten-free sandwich bread that he could eat. When we arrived, much to my dismay, I realized that I had forgotten the supplements that Jackson takes that need to be refrigerated—the probiotics, omega-3 fatty acids, and several others. I didn't worry too much about the omega-3s, but he absolutely needed the probiotics. Of course, there were none to be found in a small vacation town in the mountains.

I had never let him go without his medication and supplements and wasn't sure what type of regression he might experience. I wasn't going to risk him slipping backward in any way, so I drove to another town where I could get a cell connection and called the formulating pharmacy where I got most of Jackson's supplements. Thankfully, they had everything available and were able to overnight a package to me.

****

Back home again, Jackson went off happily to start third grade at his new school, but his enthusiasm quickly faded. He was having a hard time paying attention in class, and the teachers couldn't quite figure him out. He had been on the same low dose of ADHD medication since the first grade, so I talked to Dr. Roberts and our pediatrician about increasing the dosage. They were both in agreement, and the pediatrician gave me a new prescription.

Although I wasn't keen on giving Jackson additional drugs, I was eager to have a standard dose that no longer had to be compounded by a formulating pharmacy. As always, I gave him the higher dose on a Saturday, so I could watch for any adverse reaction. When I had tried the higher dose of ADHD medication the summer before, it had made him too anxious, but at this point, he had grown bigger physically, and he did fine with it.

I sent him to school that Monday on the new medication and got an email from his special ed teacher that afternoon. She was excited to tell me that Jackson had had a great day and that she was finally seeing the "real" Jackson and what he was capable of. The special ed teacher who worked with Jackson in the third grade was truly dedicated, but his classroom teacher had an approach I didn't particularly care for. That said, as long as Jackson was learning and went to school happily, I was fine.

Bill and I took turns lying down at night with each child to hear about their day. Jackson would tell me his innermost thoughts when I would lie down with him. I was lying in bed with Jackson one night, and I asked him if anything interesting happened in school that day.

"Well, one thing," he said, as his chin started to quiver.

"What was that?" I asked.

"When we came back from math class today," he said, "my teacher stood at the door and made us solve a multiplication problem before she'd let us go into the room. If you got it wrong, you had to go to the end of the line and couldn't go back into the classroom."

"Did you get it right?" I asked.

"No," he said. "I got it wrong three times and had to go to the end of the line each time. I was the last one to go into the classroom."

"How did that make you feel?" I asked.

"I was frustrated and just wanted to go sit at my desk, but my teacher wouldn't let me," he said.

As Jackson didn't advocate well for himself, it was with mixed feelings that I considered having him moved to another class for the rest of the school year. I didn't know if it would be disruptive for him, and I didn't want him to feel like he had failed in his third-grade class. I also didn't want him to think I was going to bail him out every time he was in a difficult situation; he needed to learn how to better stand up for himself. I didn't ask that he be moved. Unfortunately, the situation in his classroom deteriorated.

Every Monday, Jackson received a package of homework for the week. We did the appropriate assignment each night, and he turned it in the next day. One week in December, the packet didn't come home on Monday night. When I asked Jackson where it was, he said, "I left it at school."

The homework packet didn't arrive the next night either, so I sent his teacher an email asking her to remind him, and Jackson, again, assured me he'd bring it home on Wednesday. "It will be very difficult to get a week's worth of work done in one night, if it doesn't come home before Thursday," I told Jackson.

Wednesday night rolled around, and still no homework packet. I sent the following email to his classroom teacher on Wednesday evening, and this time copied the special ed teacher, as I thought his teacher might have been out for a couple of days.

I'll call the teacher Miss Hun, as in Attila the Hun.

Miss Hun,

Jackson didn't bring his homework packet for the week on Monday night (he said he forgot it) and he didn't bring it home tonight. Would you please make sure he brings it home tomorrow, so we can get it done?

Thanks very much,

Ellen

Apparently, the teacher didn't like the fact that I had copied the special ed instructor on the email, and this is what I received in return:

Mrs. Woodbriar,

Jackson was told twice to place his homework in his homework folder. I even witnessed him going into his desk to do so yesterday. I do not find it necessary to respond to emails that contain a request. You gave me a request and it was followed. If it was not, then you would have had an email. Please in the future if you have a question about something that I did or did not do, please ask me about it and not someone else.

> Jackson has been told again to place it in his folder. I dumped his desk and he put it in his folder. We have 25 witnesses to it being in his folder as it took us 10 minutes of class time to do so. We will not take this time in the future …
>
> Happy Holidays,
> Miss Hun

I'd never heard the phrase "dumping a desk" before, and I wasn't completely sure what it meant (I found out it meant that she literally picked up the desk and dumped its contents on the floor). Regardless, how thoughtful of Miss Hun to wish me happy holidays after publicly humiliating and abusing my child! I didn't respond to her email, and this next one arrived a little over an hour later.

> Mrs. Woodbriar,
>
> Upon talking with Jackson at the end of the day, I asked him why he didn't do what I had asked him to do yesterday. He said that he did but that it was his poetry packet that he placed in his homework folder. Jackson has NEVER been the student to NOT do what he is told to do. When I ask him to do something he does it … maybe not right away and sometimes I have to say it more than once, but he does do it.
>
> As he continues to get used to everything this year … please keep in mind that homework is NOT graded for a grade. He is learning how to take responsibility for himself and I think he

is doing fairly well considering where he was a few years ago. Let's continue to get him to be independent while only making a big deal out of things that need to be a big deal. I do not get stressed when students do not turn in their homework because I know that the homework I give is for practice on what is taught in class. If a child constantly misses his homework that's different, but that's not the case for Jackson. I see it in his folder and every once in a while, he decides to turn it in.

I have also found that a note helps him out ... checklists. Perhaps you can make a checklist of what he should do every morning when he comes to school and place it in his binder or agenda. (Turn in homework, give it to Miss Hun). Giving rewards and consequences for following through with the checklist can and does help him at school. Maybe it will help him with the home/school connection as well. Just something to think about.

Miss Hun

In her first email, Miss Hun had copied the special ed teacher, who had apparently pointed out Miss Hun's grave error in judgment and civility. I can only assume this second message was her veiled attempt at an apology, but it was way too little, too late. Where was the support he was supposed to be getting in the classroom? I printed both emails and immediately set up an appointment for the next day with the principal, school guidance counselor, and Jackson's special educator.

The day Miss Hun had dumped his desk, Jackson came home from school with a terrified look on his face. The minute he saw me, the tears started to roll down his cheeks. I had heard from another parent that Miss Hun had dumped out another child's desk earlier in the year because it was too messy. I ran into that same parent later that afternoon. Her daughter was in Jackson's class, and the first thing she said to me was, "Did you hear Miss Hun dumped another child's desk today? Apparently, he hadn't turned in his homework."

"It was Jackson's desk," I told her, "and that will be the last desk she ever dumps."

So now I knew that not only had she dumped out Jackson's desk, but she had also announced to the class that Jackson hadn't turned in his homework. When I lay down with Jackson that night, he relayed the entire story. Miss Hun had not only dumped the entire contents of his desk on the floor, she had thrown the desk as well. She made Jackson pick up the desk and put it back where it belonged.

The students' desks were arranged in clusters of four. The legs of the desks that abutted one another and met in the middle of the four-desk cluster were placed in a coffee can to secure them. Jackson had a hard time getting the leg of the desk back into the coffee can by himself, and no one offered to help him. I can only imagine that all the children were too terrified to move. Then, while his classmates continued to watch, he picked up all the contents of his desk from the floor and put them back.

"How did that make you feel?" I asked him.

"I was scared, and I don't want to go back to school tomorrow," he replied.

Well, no kidding! What child would want to return to such an out-of-control and abusive environment? Bill and I sat in the principal's office the next day and watched him read the exchange of emails, in dead silence, with a grim look on his face. His initial response was: "This is unacceptable."

The guidance counselor offered that not only had Miss Hun thrown the desk, but apparently it had hit another child in the foot. The principal seemed appalled not only that Miss Hun would exhibit such inappropriate behavior but that she would then show the unbelievably poor judgment to document what she had done and shoot it into cyberspace.

I made it very clear to the principal that I was two seconds away from pressing the send button that would fully inform the county's superintendent of schools. He assured Bill and me that this would never happen again and asked that I document the conversation we had in his office. I sent it to him in an email along with Miss Hun's admission of guilt. It took me more than two hours to write the email; I chose every word carefully and quoted Jackson's IEP. The response included the following key points:

- I do not believe that Jackson's IEP has been fully implemented in the classroom this year and I believe that it is the school's responsibility to implement the IEP. Having said that, I also believe that the success of any child is based on a team approach between the teacher and the parents. Jackson has three checklists at home for his home routines and should have a checklist in school to remind him of the school routine; this should be the responsibility of the teacher.
- I don't understand the hostility in the email. I simply asked that Jackson's homework come home. This was not a judgment of Miss Hun following a request but a suggestion that Jackson's support system should be implemented in Miss Hun's classroom.

- Dumping a desk and throwing it across the floor does not teach children anything other than that it is acceptable to publicly humiliate others and is not conducive to any child's development. Dumping desks as a scare tactic or pointing out any child's disability in a public forum will not help any child develop positively in any way.

- The incidents that have taken place as documented above are forming Jackson's perception of school. When asked how the incident made him feel, he said that he was scared. I asked him if he cried and he said, "I cried on the inside." He indicated to me that he was not excited to go to school the next day because he was still "scared" of what happened the day before. It was still an issue for him several days later.

- I have always copied any message to Jackson's teachers to the special educator who works with him. To address Miss Hun's concern about responding to her and not someone else, I think transparency is key to open communication, and I will continue to copy the special educator on all communication to any of Jackson's teachers.

I never heard anything back from the principal, and I knew I had been blown off. Right after the December holiday break, I was at school for something and ran into the principal. I asked him if he had received my email. He told me that he had received it, that he'd spoken with Miss Hun, and that the situation had been resolved.

The fact that she was still in the classroom told me it hadn't been resolved to my satisfaction. There had been reports of children misbehaving in her classroom, including Jackson. Of course the children were misbehaving; they didn't know how to behave in such an environment. They were being taught at home that bullying and public humiliation are unacceptable behaviors, yet these same behaviors were being modeled for them every day by their teacher.

I sent an email to the principal asking for a written response to my concerns. What I got in return assured me he had done very little about the incident. It took until January—almost five months into the school year—to fully implement Jackson's IEP, which should have been implemented within the first week of school.

My point in telling these stories is simply to illustrate that it doesn't matter how well you think things may be going in your child's life or how much respect you have for the adults with whom you trust your child every day. You can never relinquish accountability and advocacy for your child.

****

Despite the difficulties Jackson had in his classroom that year, he was able to meet life's challenges with determination and grace. He had already learned to do flips off the diving board, fish, and tube behind a boat, and was able to hike a mountain that previously would have been too challenging for him. He also decided that he wanted to learn martial arts, so Bill took him to check out the local dojo. He loved it and made a pact with his dad that he would be dedicated to it twice a week, and he would practice.

Bill signed him up, and Jackson was committed to taekwondo for several years. A month before this, I had had a conversation with Dr. Roberts about the best sports for children with ADHD. She indicated that any one-on-one event or activity where Jackson would have to get from point A to point B as fast as he could would be appropriate. Swimming or running were good examples, and she indicated that martial arts are also

213

very good, due to the amount of motor planning, discipline, and dedication they require.

We also took the kids skiing for the first time that winter. After one lesson, Jackson followed me down the slope with no trepidation but spent so much time focusing on what I was doing that he kept falling. With intense frustration, he stood at the bottom of the slope and screamed at me, loud enough for the entire resort to hear, that under no uncertain terms, I would follow *him* the next time. I didn't really have any issue with that, until he pointed both skis straight downhill and took off like a runaway locomotive. I had no choice but to follow him. I was sure if I fell at the speed with which we seemed to be moving, I'd break every bone in my body.

There was also one point on the slope where if you didn't make a hard left turn, you'd go straight over the edge of a black diamond slope, the most advanced. Now I was the one screaming, "Turn left, Jackson! Turn left!" There was no chance I was taking on a black diamond—I hadn't skied in many years, and I didn't think I could handle the challenge. As my eyes darted around the slope, I saw a member of the ski patrol standing at the turn. I assumed they were strategically placed there for situations just like this.

Remarkably, Jackson made the turn, and I didn't have to make the split-second decision, at seemingly ninety miles per hour, as to whether I should follow my child to my sure death or let the ski patrol skillfully bring his broken little body back to me. I trusted he could make the turn again and screwed up enough courage to take the slope with him one more time. It was a great weekend, and it took me only about a week to fully recover physically from the sore muscles.

****

214

Jackson had always shown an interest in music, and I had inherited my grandmother's piano the year before, so I decided it was time for both children to start piano lessons. They both took to it immediately. Abby would practice on her own, but Jackson would much rather play Wii. He was able to squeak by with his lessons without practicing; it turned out that he was somewhat capable in reading music and could pretty much sight-read whatever the teacher gave him.

Keep in mind, he was playing "Twinkle, Twinkle, Little Star," and not Chopin concertos. He played three pieces in his first recital that summer. I was nervous for both of the children, as I had never liked to play in recitals as a child, but my anxiety was unwarranted; both children played beautifully that afternoon. Listening to Jackson play the piano that day, I watched the past seven years scroll through my mind. It was almost overwhelming to think of where we had been and everything we had gone through to get to where we were that day.

Not one of the days I had watched Jackson through a one-way window as he struggled in preschool did I ever imagine I'd be sitting in someone's living room listening to him play a grand piano. Bill and I had such an array of emotions over the years since Jackson got sick; we could go from feeling we had it all together one minute to devastated the next, without any warning. Although it appeared at this point that we could have more balance in our lives, Jackson's health and our dedication to not letting him slip backward required that we remain vigilant. As Elisabeth Kubler-Ross and David Kessler say in *On Grief and Grieving: Finding the Meaning of Grief Through the Five Stages of Loss:*

> We are not accustomed to the emotional upheaval that accompanies an illness or loss ...

in order to give emotions a rest, you have to accept things as they are. You have been through a lot ... figure out what rests your emotions and do it without judgment: things like getting lost in movies, TV, music, a change of scenery, a trip away, being outdoors, or just having nothing to do.

Find what brings you some solace and lean toward it ... your life has been out of balance for some time. It will take time to find a new balance.[1]

****

Jackson had grown more than two inches and gained five pounds that year, and his behavior was indicating that he was probably due for a tune-up. We ordered a blood test to see, once again, where we were biochemically and sent the results to Dana Laake. We found Jackson's zinc, magnesium, and vitamin D3 levels to be too low for optimum function. We had also tested his copper level to make sure it wasn't being depleted from the levels of zinc he was already taking. It was fine, and we were safe in increasing the amount of zinc he was taking. Dana adjusted his supplements accordingly, and Jackson was back to himself.

At the end of third grade, Jackson's final grades were four As, five Bs, two outstandings, and two satisfactories. Surely, after our experience that year—and with Miss Hun's smoking gun just waiting in cyberspace for me to share—Jackson would be placed in a more appropriate classroom for fourth grade.

I made it crystal clear to the school that Abby, who was finishing a successful year in second grade, would not be subjected to Miss Hun's third-grade class. Apparently, I was among several parents who were not happy with Miss Hun's approach to teaching, and I was thrilled to learn that she would be taking a leave of absence for the coming school year. She never returned.

****

I hadn't seen a new or relevant resource on leaky gut in a couple of years and was looking for more current information. A friend, who had a niece with a similar diagnosis as Jackson, recommended I read *Gut and Psychology (GAP) Syndrome,* written by a British physician who had recovered her own child after a misdiagnosis of autism. I read it feverishly and wished I had found the book years earlier.

It was a wealth of information on leaky gut syndrome and the havoc it can potentially wreak, mimicking symptoms of autism, ADHD, allergies, depression, and even some of schizophrenia. I'd read this before on the Great Plains Lab website. What was new to me was the author's description of how babies' bodies are introduced to microbes:

> As far as the science knows, an unborn baby is sterile. Its body has no bacteria, viruses or fungi living in it. When the time of birth comes as the baby goes through the birth canal, it gets its first dose of microbes. Its skin, eyes, mucous membranes in the mouth and nose acquire their first micro flora. Through swallowing the liquids in the mother's vagina, the baby's digestive system gets its first population of bacteria, viruses and fungi.[2]

The book went on to explain that many mothers of children with what it calls "gut and psychology syndrome" show signs of chronic gut dysbiosis. I don't believe I have chronic gut dysbiosis, as I've never had any obvious symptoms of it, but regardless, and at Dana's suggestion, I did start taking a probiotic on a daily basis, and I also gave one to Abby.

What I did know was that, due to partial placenta previa (when the baby's placenta partially or totally covers the opening to the birth canal), Jackson was born by cesarean section and consequently never got the initial dose of microbes that babies should get. Did that start him off already depleted? Is there a significant statistical correlation between the number of babies being born by cesarean section today and the increase in autistic-like behavior, ADHD, or allergies in our children?

> There is another important factor, which makes children vulnerable—the toxic load which the child is born with. What is it? For years we believed that the placenta in a pregnant woman protects the fetus from any toxins which the woman might have in her body. Recent studies show that we were wrong. The fetus accumulates most toxins, which the mother is exposed to … Depending on how toxic the mother is during pregnancy different babies are born with a different toxic load.[3]

Did Jackson start his life at a disadvantage? Do all children with autism, ADHD, or allergies start their lives this way?

The most common condition that Dr. Campbell-McBride sees in siblings of children with severe leaky gut are allergies like eczema and asthma, which are the result of a malfunctioning immune system. Abby had eczema and a mild form of asthma, both of which she outgrew, and she had also been born by cesarean section. Dr. Campbell-McBride had many of the same questions I did as she treated her child and those in her clinic.

> What underlying problem are we missing in our children which makes them susceptible to asthma, eczema, allergies, dyspraxia, dyslexia, behavioral problems, ADHD and autism in different combinations? ... To answer all of these questions we have to look at one factor, which unites all these patients in a clinical setting. This factor is the state of their digestive system ... Children with GAP Syndrome often fall into the gap—the gap in our medical knowledge. As a result, they do not receive appropriate treatment.[4]

Although it took time to find the right team of doctors and treatment, I am eternally grateful that Jackson did receive appropriate treatment. He continued to grow intellectually, emotionally, and physically throughout third grade. His resilience allowed him to absorb the lessons from all his experiences, both positive and negative.

As I lay in bed with Jackson one night that summer, he asked me, "Mommy, who is God's father?"

"I don't know," I responded. "Who do you think is God's father?"

He thought for a moment. "Maybe he was the first person in the universe, or maybe he was from some huge energy force in space."

"I don't think anyone has a better answer than that," I said.

Just before he fell asleep, I asked, "Jackson, what do you think is particularly special in your life?"

He lay quietly by my side for a few minutes. Then he said, "Mom, everything is special in my life."

CHAPTER 14

LESSONS LEARNED

· · · · · · · · · · ·

Seventeen years ago, I was at a point where I didn't know if my son was going to live. I didn't know if he would degenerate in front of my eyes from a malignant form of epilepsy or a neurodegenerative disorder; if he was autistic; if he would ever have a friend; if he would someday be able to think clearly enough to string together a coherent sentence; or if he would ever again be able to run, jump, and play.

Those years were weighted with stress, anxiety, fear, and guilt—on top of the pressures of everyday life, parenting, and work. It is wearying looking backward, but at this point, there's no reason to do so. Jackson's recovery is truly extraordinary, and we now move forward every day. Things change more slowly, and life is more predictable.

Bill and I have learned so many lessons over the past seventeen years, in multiple aspects of our lives. The lessons that stand out are mostly associated with advocating for your children, yourself, and your relationships. We didn't learn them alone, and we feel a responsibility to pass them on in the hope that they might help others.

Under this umbrella of advocacy, the lessons that I think would be most helpful to any family relate to recognizing siblings; developing confidence and self-esteem; supporting academic endeavors; understanding the important contribution that movement and exercise make to health; monitoring of health and new research on a regular basis; preparing for the future; and remembering your own life.

Siblings Deserve Recognition Too

Abby's role in Jackson's recovery has been paramount. Without realizing it, she's been the best therapy that Jackson could have had. I think she knew exactly what she was doing when she came to be his sister, and if we'd had to pay for what she's done for Jackson, we couldn't have afforded her. She has been a speech, occupational, and physical therapist all rolled into one. She's also challenged Jackson's social skills by being his confidante as well as his sparring partner.

Abby demanded engaged communication and answers to her questions when Jackson still struggled to access his language. She expected no less of him physically than what she was able to do herself. If she wanted to race, then he needed to run. If she wanted to swing, then he needed to learn to pump his legs. At this writing, Abby is seventeen and a senior in high school. Jackson is two years older and a college freshman. She remains demanding of him, and it's engaging to watch how their relationship has grown.

Like most older brothers (based on my own experience), Jackson likes to have the upper hand physically—he holds her down and tickles her, likes to stick his dirty socks in her face, and generally picks at her until he gets the desired reaction. I always smile as I listen to the laughing, protesting, and squealing, because just a few years ago, there was none. Through the countless arguments over the television remote or who was going to sit next to whom, they've both learned semi appropriate reciprocal behavior.

Over the years, I've tried to plan one-on-one activities with Abby. Now, at seventeen, she'd rather be out with her friends than spend time with Bill and me—age-appropriate behavior but slightly painful, nonetheless. At this point, time together has to be on her terms. When she's willing to talk, I try to be there to listen.

Confidence and Self-Esteem Are Critical to Development

From many perspectives, middle school is one of those miserable rites of passage that we all must endure. I'm not sure I've ever met an American child or parent who actually enjoyed middle school. It's a period of transition, social development, and growth, and a struggle for independence. Jackson is no exception; he didn't skate through middle school unscathed. Although he had a small group of friends, he compared himself to more popular children and wanted to be part of a bigger group or team. His lack of confidence helped make him a target to a few bullies, which undermined his self-esteem. He also felt the pressure of getting good grades.

The mean-spirited behaviors that can be displayed by both boys and girls seem to be second to none throughout the school-age years. I don't think Jackson was made fun of any more often than any other child, but he seemed to lack the self-confidence to rise above it. I did discover that some of the boys that harassed or bullied him had developmental differences of their own to deal with and were trying to establish a pecking order among their group.

One boy would follow Jackson down the hall saying, "Hi, Jackson. Hi, Jackson," and when Jackson would finally acknowledge him and say hello, he'd say, "Fuck you, Jackson!"

This continually recurring behavior upset Jackson to the point we sought the advice of a therapist to give him pointers on how to handle the situation and potential others like it. I also talked with the school guidance counselor to see if she could intervene without being blatantly obvious. Through observation in the hallway, she did to try to catch the child in the act, but she never witnessed an encounter.

But it taught us the importance of additional growth in Jackson's ongoing development: self-advocacy, which comes with self-esteem. Our best advice to Jackson ended up being that the boy obviously had issues of his own, and the best approach was to ignore him. If he couldn't get the reaction he wanted, he'd probably stop; eventually, he did.

Middle school also came with crushes and unrequited love. Although it's sometimes difficult to watch your child go through these awkward stages of growth, Jackson was doing exactly what he was supposed to be doing when he was supposed to be doing it.

Academic Support Is Essential to a Child's Success

In contrast to Jackson's experience in the third grade, he went on to have some of the most impressive elementary, middle, and high school teachers I've met. He hasn't needed consistent occupational therapy since the second grade, and he hasn't had speech therapy since the fourth grade.

By the time Jackson reached middle school, he no longer needed help doing his schoolwork. He mastered most concepts along with his peers. But he continued to have significant executive functioning difficulties, because of ADHD, and a slower processing speed than typical peers. He did, therefore, need help staying on task and getting his work done.

In middle school, he had a case manager: a special educator who regularly checks in with a child with an IEP, to make sure they're progressing on track and to provide support where needed. She seemed genuinely interested in all the children she taught. She offered to let Jackson come to her classroom three days per week after school to get his homework done. Occasionally, she helped him with a concept, but mostly she provided the structure that he needed after school to get his work done.

Jackson no longer wanted help from Bill or me—and we were grateful to have someone to help us. By the time we got home from work each day, it was late, we were all tired, and Jackson's ADHD medication would have worn off. It was close to impossible to get any work done at that point, so the case manager's solution worked out well. Jackson was also able to take a late school bus to our neighborhood, so transportation didn't become a logistical factor for two working parents.

But ninth grade presented a struggle to keep up academically. Many assignments were completed but not turned in, and some were never completed. Often Jackson's study guides for tests were not done, yet his test scores were high. When I asked Jackson why he didn't do the study guides, which were worth a lot of points toward his grades, he would answer, "Why should I do the study guide? I got an A on the test."

I had to agree that he had a point. But zeros on the study guides were having an adverse effect on his overall grades, and so were the missing homework assignments. Jackson clearly needed more direction after school, but Bill and I could not provide it ourselves. Jackson's As and Bs started to fall as he transitioned to the higher demands of high school.

An after-school program at his high school, staffed by teachers, offered help to any child who needed it and was willing to ask for it. Jackson refused to go, saying, "That's where all the kids with ADHD and autism go."

We reminded him that he too had ADHD, but he didn't want to be labeled. When he was younger, so many children had made fun of him or made comments—particularly after the desk-dumping incident—and the memories were strong. He didn't want to be associated with the treatment he had painfully discovered often comes with a learning difference. He wanted to be like his typical peers—and at that point, for the most part, he was.

By the winter of his freshman year, it was clear that we needed to hire a tutor. I advertised with the special education departments in three local universities as well as with tutors listed as available through a school for children with learning differences. Out of four institutions, I got one reply. So, without any process of elimination, we hired her. She had worked with Jackson for about four months, when we had an appointment with Dr. Roberts.

Jackson opened up, telling Dr. Roberts that he really didn't enjoy working with the tutor—hated it, actually. Bill and I already had sensed strongly that the tutor wasn't the right fit. They had nothing in common, and the tutor didn't have the breadth of experience that we needed to help Jackson with all subjects. She mostly focused on English and writing, which was helpful but not enough. When I called to let her go, she sounded relieved. I think she was in over her head with some subjects and knew she couldn't provide the executive-functioning support that Jackson needed.

Timing would have it that a friend's son, Zach, had just graduated from college with a degree in engineering. He didn't have a permanent job yet, and he could help Jackson with all his subjects. Jackson was way behind in his Introduction to Engineering class, and Zach helped him catch up. In fact, he helped him catch up in all his classes, and Jackson ended the year on a much higher note than we had expected in February. Zach moved on to a great job in his own field, and we were able to hire another wonderful tutor and executive coach, found through an agency. She would see Jackson through his senior year and help Abby, when needed, as well.

Movement and Exercise Contribute to Overall Health

It is established that exercise has a positive effect on cognition, ability to focus, motor planning, and mood. As Jackson continued to recover and feel stronger physically, he wanted to learn some of the sports he had been too sick to participate in when he was younger.

We supported him in every venture, going through several years of exposure to taekwondo, diving, golf, basketball, tennis, fishing, and skiing. Taekwondo and skiing were the only two sports that really stuck with Jackson. He joined the ski club in the seventh grade, and continued through high school to ski every Friday night in January and February at a not-too-distant resort with his school club. He went on to achieve first-degree black belt status in taekwondo, in the summer of 2015, and made a goal of becoming a fourth-degree black belt, so we would have to call him "Master."

With the beginning of ninth grade, he developed a love for baseball; his history teacher was the baseball coach, and I think that's where his interest originated. He came home from school one afternoon and told me that he'd signed up for the junior varsity baseball team tryouts. I replied, "That's great, but you do realize you've never played baseball."

To which he replied, "I played T-ball when I was six."

I was pretty confident that one year of T-ball at six would not make him a high school baseball player, but he was determined.

Bill found a baseball organization that offered coaching to all levels of ability and signed Jackson up for lessons. He went two to three times per week from fall until spring, did all the high school winter workouts with the others trying out for the team, and no longer had time for taekwondo. He was cut from the baseball team on the last day of tryouts. Although he was disappointed, he had a great attitude. He said that he wanted to play in a recreational league, so that he could get better and try out again his sophomore year.

Jackson played in the local recreational league in the spring of his freshman year. He went to Ripken Baseball Camp that summer and played again in a fall recreational league as a sophomore. He participated in high school baseball workouts in the winter of his sophomore year but, again, was cut from the team.

He didn't give up; he continued in the recreational league, attended baseball camp, and volunteered at a different baseball camp over the summer between sophomore and junior years to teach younger children how to play the game. In his junior year, Jackson signed up for weightlifting every day in PE class to build his strength. In a determined attempt to be part of the high school baseball team, Jackson tried out again in the spring of his junior year. Sadly, he was cut.

When Jackson didn't make the baseball team his sophomore year, he had decided to play on the school's allied softball team. Two of his teachers coached that team, and they were very persuasive in convincing him to join. Allied teams have the option to be composed of 50 percent students with disabilities and 50 percent without; however, the students without a disability cannot have played on a junior varsity or varsity team in the past. Allied softball is played indoors in a gym with some different rules than regulation softball, but the basics are the same. Jackson ended up being the pitcher and team captain and won the award at the end of the season for team sportsmanship.

What makes Bill and me happy is that with all the workouts, some twice per day, Jackson stays in good shape physically, and that greatly contributes to his overall health. In addition, his love of baseball has led to an even stronger father-son bond, as they enjoy watching and attending professional baseball games together.

Monitoring Health and New Research Is Ongoing

Jackson hasn't had a seizure, or visible seizure activity, in sixteen years as of this writing, and he has been off seizure medication for twelve. He also doesn't show signs of an overgrowth of yeast, clostridia, or any other bacteria, and he no longer needs Nystatin or an antifungal. On the rare occasion he requires an antibiotic, he no longer experiences a regression.

However, as a person with a significant medical history, monitoring is key, regardless of how healthy Jackson may seem or appear.

When Jackson reached eighth grade, I could no longer keep an eye on his eating habits outside of the house. In consultation with Dr. Roberts, we slowly introduced gluten back into his diet. There was no irritability, no gastric distress, no brain fog, and ultimately no visible effect of changing his diet. We then started introducing casein, also with no physical side effects, emotional irritability, or regression. Jackson's diet had been gluten- and dairy-free for a full ten years; it appeared that his gastrointestinal tract had healed enough that he could now handle foods containing these hard-to-digest substances. We'd reached another monumental milestone in his recovery.

Between nutritional supplements, ADHD medication, and allergy meds, Jackson was taking close to thirty pills daily. Although it was becoming increasingly more difficult to get him to take those pills, Dr. Roberts and Dana Laake recommended that they continue until he was through puberty and had finished growing—probably at least through age eighteen, as some boys have an additional growth spurt between seventeen and eighteen (my brother and I both grew through our eighteenth year). This would ensure he got the full nutrition that he needed to function optimally.

When Jackson was fifteen, it had been some time since his last tune-up. He'd grown significantly, and we wanted to ensure he continued to be biochemically balanced and nutritionally sound, so we decided to repeat blood, stool, and urine tests.

The test results showed that we needed to tweak a few things. But for the most part, Jackson was doing well. The nutrition evaluation didn't show any results that were a high need, but he was a bit borderline on some antioxidants, specifically vitamin C and CoQ10 (a powerful antioxidant that is synthesized in the body and contained in cell membranes and is also essential for energy production and pH regulation), B vitamins, and minerals. Dana increased these in his supplements. His yeast and fungal dysbiosis markers had remained the same for the past two years and were negative.

One area of concern was that he had an oxidative stress marker—meaning his body appeared unable to adequately reduce the negative effect of free radicals. An increase in antioxidants would be most helpful, and Dr. Roberts thought this would resolve with the additional CoQ10 and B vitamins. Thankfully, at this point, Jackson showed no signs of toxicity from the heavy metals (mercury and aluminum) he had shown earlier in his life.

It was agreed that the dose of ADHD medication Jackson was taking was still quite low and could be increased. We were able to do so just before the end of his freshman year. As in the past, the new dosage boosted not only his executive functioning ability but also his processing speed.

Although I feel as though I have a depth of knowledge in leaky gut syndrome, some types of seizure activity, and nutritional health, I'm still left with many of the same questions I had when I started this book. What were the variables that led to the leaky gut that potentially caused the regression

Jackson experienced over a four-month period, the irritability he exhibited, the sixty to eighty seizures he endured each day, and the autistic-like behavior he developed?

Was it the milk allergy he had as an infant? Seasonal allergies, mostly to pollen and leaf mold, resulting in ongoing sinus and ear infections followed by multiple courses of antibiotics? Preservatives in vaccines? Other viruses? Exposure to toxins from pollutants? Was it because he was blond and green-eyed, a result of every recessive gene in our family's gene pool? Could it have been an underlying autoimmune deficiency? Stress from the birth of his new sister? The fact that he was delivered by cesarean section? Or a combination of all of the above?

At this writing, there is so much more research available on gut issues than when we started this journey. Yet I would ask leading research or medical institutions to prove me right, or even wrong. However, at this point, I believe the latter would be difficult.

There was no one pill or medication that helped Jackson. There's no one pill to help medically complex children with similar symptoms and behavior. There's also no one pill to help autistic people who suffer with some of their symptoms or behavior. For these reasons, I don't anticipate major pharmaceutical companies funding or sponsoring related research.

My hypothesis continues to be that some children with autistic-like behaviors are not autistic and are not receiving the full breadth of intervention that potentially could help them recover. As Dr. Michael J. Goldberg, MD, says in *The Myth of Autism: How a Misunderstood Epidemic Is Destroying Our Children*: "What often may seem good enough under the guise of 'autism,' 'ADHD,' or other 'LD' is not really nearly good enough if one starts thinking they began with a normal, or above-normal child."[1]

What parent would want *less* for their child?

Live in the Present but Prepare for the Future

During the spring of Jackson's freshman year and before his annual review, Bill and I thought it would be a good idea to repeat a neuropsychology evaluation. He had not had an evaluation of that nature since the first grade. Now almost sixteen, he'd grown and obviously developed significantly, and we wanted to make sure that his IEP addressed his current needs and provided appropriate support in high school. Mostly, we needed to obtain an update on how his brain-mediated abilities and skills were developing as he moved toward adulthood.

Jackson would also need an updated report as he neared College Board testing and the college application process. On the recommendation of a friend, we approached a different neuropsychologist, who had treated all three of her children with ADHD. This neuropsychologist also specializes in cognitive behavioral therapy for people with ADHD. According to the nonprofit organization Children and Adults with Attention Deficit Hyperactivity Disorder (CHADD), the national resource on ADHD:

> Programs that address executive dysfunction fall into the category of cognitive-behavioral therapy because they impart more adaptive cognitions about how to go about planning, organizing, etc. and also impart more effective behavioral skills. An example of an adaptive cognition is the self-instruction to break down

complex or unpleasant tasks into manageable parts. Examples of behavioral skills are using a planner regularly and implementing a filing system.

Positive thoughts and positive behaviors reinforce each other; as the person becomes more effective in managing time, s/he comes to have more positive beliefs and cognitions about the self, and these in turn help to generate and maintain more adaptive behaviors.[2]

We completed the evaluation over a three-day period in March 2016 and waited for the report, which we received in May.

Jackson was fifteen years and ten months old at the time of the evaluation. It confirmed the findings from the evaluation completed in 2008: "Jackson initially presents as a bright, healthy, well developed, polite, somewhat shy, inhibited and introversive adolescent male."

The evaluation indicated that Jackson showed improvement in his performance in general cognitive ability at a high-average level. However, it went on to indicate continued areas of concern that seem to contribute to Jackson's challenges, for example:

Difficulty sustaining his attention to tasks that he must complete that are not of interest to him or he perceives as tedious or boring.

Slowed speed of information processing that results in it taking Jackson significantly longer than his peers to complete work.

> Difficulty feeling comfortable in situations where he will or could be evaluated by others ... including managing some of his social anxiety and fear of judgement.

The development of executive functioning components has a more profound effect on an individual's ability to achieve success in school and life than most other areas in one's cognitive profile, including intelligence. The psychologist included that "working to accommodate and then facilitate the development of executive function is a long-term project that requires effort from the parents, teachers, tutors, learning specialists, and individuals themselves."

As with the previous evaluation, we knew all this, but we needed current testing to make sure that Jackson's IEP was continuing to meet his needs. It was. The current IEP focuses on completing work and turning it in on time, planning skills, the need to better advocate for himself, and adding detail to his writing. He can complete his academic work without support, but he needs help with strategies around executive function (i.e., planning) to make sure it gets done. In fact, because Jackson does so well in school academically, he took one honors and two advanced placement (AP) classes as a junior. He planned to take three more AP classes his senior year.

We started implementing strategies related to "self-determination, self-advocacy, and academic skills,"[3] to better prepare him for college. I read several books on readying a student with ADHD to move out of the house and become more successful at independence, including *Ready for Take-off: Preparing Your Teen With ADHD or LD for College; ADD and the College Student; A Guide for High School and College Students with Attention Deficit Disorder;* and *Making the Grade with A+DD: A Student's Guide to Succeeding in College with Attention Deficit Disorder.* We visited colleges the spring of Jackson's junior year and throughout that summer in search of the right fit for Jackson. He was looking for an environmental science program. We've come such a very long way from the little boy who sat on his preschool teacher's lap wearing a weighted vest and struggling to form a sentence.

Remember Your Own Life

It's 2020 and spring again. Jackson just finished his freshman year in college, and Abby is graduating from high school. We're recovering as a family. The daffodils, tulips, and forsythia have all bloomed, the trees are leafing, and once again I can feel the warmth of the sun. Someone once told me that no matter what life may hand you, "God always brings spring." It doesn't matter at what stage you are in your journey, or what you may have to endure; if you allow it, and are open to it, spring will eventually come.

As the children have grown and Jackson has recovered, the last few years have allowed Bill and me the time to focus a bit more on ourselves. Bill has been able to run with more regularity and I signed up with a personal trainer. We have a few more date nights but not as many as some of the couples we know. We've turned into homebodies and prefer a movie in front of our own TV or preparing a quiet dinner with friends or family.

Bill and I were both still working about sixty hours per week when Jackson was a sophomore and Abby a freshman in high school. Like so many parents, "trying to do it all, have it all, and give it all to my children, I realized that in fact, I was setting a pace that left us scattered and exhausted."[4] We decided we'd missed enough of our children's childhoods, and I was able to retire from corporate executive life in the summer of 2017.

With two children still at home, life filled in quickly. I now spend my time taking care of my home and family, catching up with friends (some with whom I'd lost contact), working on the projects that I'd started but hadn't finished (including this book), and trying to be kind and patient with myself. I taught Jackson to drive, and he now has his license, which comes with additional independence. I loved attending both kids' sports events and especially enjoyed shuttling them and their team members while listening to the chatter in the car. I heard so much about what was going on in their lives that way. Over the past ten years, I've learned to meditate and to try to stay grounded, and I now don't rush unless I have to. One downside is that I'm now typically late for everything, and my family complains bitterly about it! But I'd rather be stress-free and relaxed than compulsively on time, as long as I'm not grossly inconveniencing anyone.

The experiences I've shared in this book and the lessons I've learned from them have led me through a metamorphosis of unimaginable significance. The trivial things that once consumed me are no longer of any consequence. The more simply I can live my life, the better, and "complicated" doesn't impress me. I dream of the day when I have the time to remove the clutter from my life and my home, and with my recent retirement, I hope it has arrived. I don't have strong feelings about what my children grow up to be, as long as they are healthy, happy, strong, safe, and loved; can live their lives the way they choose; and can sustain themselves.

My favorite Saturday night is sitting in our family room by the fire in the winter, or on our screened porch in the summer, enjoying the flowers in my garden and the goldfinches on the bird feeder. Maybe that's all the energy I have left. But I sincerely feel cheated if I miss any weekend nights at home when my family is all together. There are no fixed routines or deadlines on Friday and Saturday nights, no homework must be done, nor a bedtime enforced. For the time being, no one is sick, and everyone can breathe deeply again and enjoy one another.

That kind of life may sound boring to some. But I'm content with what William and I have achieved—through our determination and with the help of so many others. Like everyone else, I have no idea what the future will bring, but I do know that if and when we face future challenges, we'll have the resilience to cope with them.

I go back to my opening words: I told this story with the hope of helping even one other parent, physician, teacher, or therapist to look beyond the obvious and dig as deeply as needs be to help recover a child. I hope the information in this book has offered some new and enlightening perspectives to those who work with, but have not raised, a medically complex child. I also hope it will be a resource and provide reference for those parents who are raising a child with differences.

All children deserve unconditional love and care, and I'm thankful every day that Jackson and Abby came to be mine.

GLOSSARY

· · · · · · · · · · ·

The following terms are found within the text of *Lessons from a Complex Child*. Some of the following definitions and explanations have been taken from references within the text of this book. However, the majority come from the National Institutes of Health (NIH) US National Library of Medicine, which is within the public domain.[5] Most of the following definitions and descriptions are excerpts from the full information provided on the library's website.

5-hydroxyindoleacetic acid (5-HIAA): The primary metabolite of serotonin, a chemical substance (neurotransmitter) that transmits messages between nerve cells. Serotonin is produced as needed by the nervous system, mainly the brain, but also special cells in the bronchial tubes (lungs) and gastrointestinal (GI) tract. It helps transmit nerve impulses and constrict blood vessels, participates in the wake-sleep cycle, and affects mood. Large quantities of serotonin and 5-HIAA may be produced, however, by some carcinoid tumors. See "carcinoid tumors."

absence seizure: This type of seizure affects the whole brain and usually only lasts a few seconds. During the seizure, a person may have a staring spell, be unaware of his or her surroundings, suddenly stop talking or moving, or have small changes in muscle movements. These types of seizures have also been known as petit mal.

acupressure: A method in Traditional Chinese Medicine (TCM) that involves placing pressure on an area of your body, using fingers or another device, to help restore health. It is similar to acupuncture. In TCM, acupressure and acupuncture work by changing the messages (such as pain) that nerves send to your brain.

adenosine triphosphate (ATP): A substance present in all living cells that provides energy for many metabolic processes and is involved in making ribonucleic acid (RNA). The primary function of RNA is protein synthesis within a cell.

aluminum: A metallic element that is found combined with other elements in the earth's crust. It is also found in small amounts in soil, water, and many foods. It is used in medicine and dentistry and in many products, such as foil, cans, pots and pans, airplanes, siding, and roofs. High levels of aluminum in the body can be harmful. Aluminum accumulates in the kidneys, brain, lungs, liver, and thyroid, where it competes with calcium for absorption and can affect skeletal mineralization. In infants, this can slow growth. Animal models have linked aluminum exposure to mental impairments.

anaerobic: Indicates "without oxygen." The term has many uses in medicine. Anaerobic bacteria are germs that can survive and grow where there is no oxygen. For example, it can thrive in human tissue that is injured and does not have oxygen-rich blood flowing to it. Infections like tetanus and gangrene are caused by anaerobic bacteria. Anaerobic infections typically cause abscesses (buildups of pus) and death of tissue. Many anaerobic bacteria produce enzymes that destroy tissue or sometimes release potent toxins.

antihistamine: Drugs that treat allergy symptoms. Even though they do not cure allergies, colds, or the flu, they provide welcome relief for at least some of the discomforts of seasonal allergies and upper respiratory infections.

antioxidant: The body ... makes molecules that fight free radicals. We also extract free-radical fighters from food. These molecules are typically called "antioxidants." There are hundreds, probably thousands, of different substances that can act as antioxidants. The most familiar ones are vitamin C, vitamin E, beta-carotene, and other related carotenoids, along with the minerals selenium and manganese. They're joined by glutathione, CoQ10, lipoic acid, flavonoids, phenols, polyphenols, phytoestrogens, and many more. See "free radicals."

atonic seizures: Cause a loss of normal muscle tone, which often leads the affected person to fall down or drop the head involuntarily.

attention deficit hyperactivity disorder (ADHD): A disorder that makes it difficult for a person to pay attention and control impulsive behaviors. He or she may also be restless and almost constantly active ... Although the symptoms of ADHD begin in childhood, ADHD can continue through adolescence and adulthood. Even though hyperactivity tends to improve as a child becomes a teen, problems with inattention, disorganization, and poor impulse control often continue through the teen years and into adulthood ... People with ADHD show an ongoing pattern of three different types of symptoms: Difficulty paying attention (inattention), being overactive (hyperactivity), and acting without thinking (impulsivity). These symptoms get in the way of functioning or development.

autism spectrum disorder (ASD): A neurological and developmental disorder that begins early in childhood and lasts throughout a person's life. It affects how a person acts and interacts with others, communicates, and learns. It includes what used to be known as Asperger syndrome and pervasive developmental disorders. It is called a "spectrum" disorder because people with ASD can have a range of symptoms. People with ASD might have problems talking with you, or they might not look you in the eye when you talk to them. They may also have restricted interests and repetitive behaviors. They may spend a lot of time putting things in order, or they may say the same sentence again and again. They may often seem to be in their own world. The causes of ASD are not known. Research suggests that both genes and environment play important roles.

bifidobacterium: A group of bacteria that normally live in the intestines. They can be grown outside the body and then taken by mouth as medicine. Bifidobacteria are commonly used for diarrhea, constipation, an intestinal disorder called irritable bowel syndrome, for preventing the common cold or flu, and lots of other conditions. See "irritable bowel syndrome."

bioflavonoid: Some articles claim that flavonoids have powerful antioxidant properties, and these are becoming very popular because they have many health-promoting effects. Some of the activities potentially attributed to flavonoids include antiallergic, anticancer, antioxidant, anti-inflammatory, and antiviral. The flavonoid quercetin is known for its seeming ability to relieve hay fever, eczema, sinusitis, and asthma; for reducing the risk for cancer; and for protection against osteoporosis. Consumption of red wine (in moderation), red grape juice, grape skin, and grape seeds have also been linked to health benefits, as they contain bioflavonoids.

C. difficile: *C. difficile* toxin is a harmful substance produced by the bacterium *clostridium* difficile (*C. difficile*). This infection is a common cause of diarrhea after antibiotic use.

candida: A yeast (fungus) that causes mild disease, but in immunocompromised individuals it may cause life-threatening illness. The fungus candida is normally found on and in the body in small amounts. It is present on the skin and in the mouth, as well as in the intestinal tract and genital area. Most of the time, candida does not cause any symptoms. When these organisms overgrow, they can cause infections (candidiasis), which sometimes can become chronic. If the fungus enters the bloodstream, the infection can spread to other parts of the body.

carcinogens: Substances and exposures that can lead to cancer are called carcinogens. Cancer is caused by changes in a cell's DNA—its genetic blueprint. Some of these changes may be inherited from our parents. Others may be caused by outside exposures, which are often referred to as environmental factors. Carcinogens do not cause cancer in every case, all the time.

carcinoid tumors: Slow-growing noncancerous or cancerous neuroendocrine masses that can form in the GI tract, especially in the appendix and in the lungs.

casein: A protein found in milk that is particularly difficult for some to digest. It may also cause allergic reaction in those who are sensitive to it.

casomorphin: The opiate-like by-products from casein (dairy). It is speculated that some children often crave this food group due to its ability to create this opiate-like effect.

computed tomography (CT or CAT) scan: A type of imaging that uses special x-ray equipment to make cross-sectional pictures of the body. During a CT scan, you lie still on a table. The table slowly passes through the center of a large x-ray machine. The test is painless. Some tests use a contrast dye, which makes parts of the body show up better in the image.

celiac disease: An immune disease in which people can't eat gluten because it will damage their small intestine. Celiac disease affects each person differently. Symptoms may occur in the digestive system or in other parts of the body. One person might have diarrhea and abdominal pain, while another person may be irritable or depressed. Irritability is one of the most common symptoms in children. See "gluten."

central nervous system: Composed of the brain and spinal cord. The brain and spinal cord serve as the main processing center for the entire nervous system. They control all the workings of the body.

Child Find: A component of Individuals with Disabilities Education Act (IDEA) that requires states to identify, locate, and evaluate all children with disabilities, age birth to twenty-one, who are in need of early intervention or special education services. The Child Find website is mainly focused on Part C of the IDEA, the Early Intervention Program for Infants and Toddlers with Disabilities.

Crohn's disease: Causes inflammation of the digestive system. It is one of a group of diseases called inflammatory bowel disease. Crohn's can affect any area from the mouth to the anus. It often affects the lower part of the small intestine called the ileum. The cause of Crohn's disease is unknown. It may be due to an abnormal reaction by the body's immune system. It also seems to run in some families. It most commonly starts between the ages of thirteen and thirty.

clostridia: Bacterium commonly found in the intestinal tract but that, under the right circumstances, such as after or during antibiotics therapy, can be the cause of enterocolitis. See "*C. difficile.*"

cognitive behavioral therapy (CBT): Cognitive behavioral therapy is a psychosocial intervention that is the most widely used evidence-based practice for improving mental health. Guided by empirical research, CBT focuses on the development of personal coping strategies that target solving current problems and changing unhelpful patterns in cognitions, behaviors, and emotional regulation.

CoQ10: A powerful antioxidant that is synthesized in the body and contained in cell membranes and is also essential for energy production and pH regulation.

developmental pediatrician: A pediatrician devoted to the care of children with delays, learning differences, or disabilities.

dysbiosis: A disturbance or imbalance in a biological system— for example, changes in the types and numbers of bacteria in the gut, which may lead to developing different diseases.

Do Not Resuscitate (DNR): A medical order written by a doctor. It instructs health care providers not to do cardiopulmonary resuscitation (CPR) if a patient's breathing stops or if the patient's heart stops beating. A DNR order is created, or set up, before an emergency occurs. A DNR order allows you to choose whether or not you want CPR in an emergency. It is specific about CPR. It does not have instructions for other treatments, such as pain medicine, other medicines, or nutrition. The doctor writes the order only after talking about it with the patient (if possible), the proxy, or the patient's family.

E. coli: E. coli is the name of a type of bacteria that lives in the intestines. Most types of E. coli are harmless. However, some types can make you sick and cause diarrhea. The worst type of E. coli causes bloody diarrhea and can sometimes cause kidney failure and even death. These problems are most likely to occur in children and in adults with weak immune systems. You can get E. coli infections by eating foods containing the bacteria.

electroencephalogram (EEG): A test used to find problems related to electrical activity of the brain. An EEG tracks and records brain wave patterns. Small metal discs with thin wires (electrodes) are placed on the scalp and then send signals to a computer to record the results. Normal electrical activity in the brain makes a recognizable pattern. Through an EEG, doctors can look for abnormal patterns that indicate seizures and other problems.

enteric nervous system (ENS): Autonomic nervous system within the walls of the digestive tract. The ENS regulates digestion and the muscle contractions that eliminate solid waste.

epilepsy: Epilepsy is a disorder of the brain. People who have epilepsy have electrical activity in the brain that is not normal, causing seizures. There are different types of seizures. In some cases, a seizure may cause jerking, uncontrolled movements and loss of consciousness. In other cases, seizures cause only a period of confusion, a staring spell, or muscle spasms. Epilepsy is also called a "seizure disorder." A single seizure is not considered epilepsy. People who have epilepsy have repeated episodes of seizures. Epilepsy is not a mental illness, and it is not a sign of low intelligence. It is also not contagious. Seizures do not normally cause brain damage. Between seizures, a person with epilepsy is no different from anyone else. Epilepsies have many possible causes, but for up to half of people with epilepsy, a cause is not known. In other cases, the epilepsies are clearly linked to genetic factors, developmental brain abnormalities, infection, traumatic brain injury, stroke, brain tumors, or other identifiable problems. Anything that disturbs the normal pattern of neuronal activity—from illness to brain damage to abnormal brain development—can lead to seizures.

facultative anaerobes: A microorganism that can grow in the presence of air or under conditions of reduced oxygen.

fatty acid oxidation: A multistep process that occurs within mitochondria to break down (metabolize) fats and convert them into energy.

folic acid: A B vitamin that helps the body make healthy new cells. Everyone needs folic acid. Getting enough folic acid before and during pregnancy can prevent major birth defects of a baby's brain or spine.

free radicals: Highly unstable molecules that are naturally formed when you exercise and when your body converts food into energy. Your body can also be exposed to free radicals from a variety of environmental sources, such as cigarette smoke, air pollution, and sunlight. Free radicals can cause oxidative stress, a process that can trigger cell damage. See "oxidative stress."

gliadorphin: The opiate-like by-products from gluten (wheat, barley, rye). It is speculated that some children often crave this food group due to their ability to create this opiate-like effect.

glutathione: An antioxidant that is important to the normal functioning of the intestine and lungs. Glutathione levels have been shown to be lower in people with cystic fibrosis, and oral glutathione may improve growth and decrease gut inflammation in children. It is capable of preventing damage to important cellular components caused by reactive oxygen species such as free radicals and heavy metals.

gluten: A protein found in wheat, rye, and barley. It may also be in other products like vitamins and supplements, hair and skin products, toothpastes, and lip balm. Gluten is difficult for some to digest and may cause an allergic reaction in those who are sensitive to it.

histamine: A substance in the body that causes allergy symptoms. Mast cells release histamine when an allergen is encountered. The histamine response can produce sneezing, itching, hives, and watery eyes.

HPHPA: A metabolite of tyrosine produced by gastrointestinal bacteria of *clostridia* species including *C. difficile*.

immunology: A branch of biomedical science that covers the study of immune systems in all organisms. An autoimmune disease is a condition arising from an abnormal immune response to a normal body part. There are at least eighty types of autoimmune diseases, such as asthma or arthritis. Nearly any body part can be involved. Common symptoms include low-grade fever and feeling tired. Often symptoms come and go.

irritable bowel syndrome (IBS): A problem that affects the large intestine. It can cause abdominal cramping, bloating, and a change in bowel habits. Some people with the disorder have constipation. Some have diarrhea. Others go back and forth between the two. Although IBS can cause a great deal of discomfort, it does not harm the intestines. IBS is common. It affects about twice as many women as men and is most often found in people younger than forty-five years. No one knows the exact cause of IBS. There is no specific test for it.

lactobacillus: These are friendly bacteria that normally live in the digestive, urinary, and genital systems without causing disease. There are lots of different species of lactobacillus. Lactobacillus is also in some fermented foods like yogurt and in dietary supplements. Lactobacillus is taken by mouth to treat and prevent diarrhea, including infectious types such as rotaviral diarrhea in children and traveler's diarrhea. It is also taken by mouth to prevent and treat diarrhea associated with using antibiotics.

Landau-Kleffner: A rare malady in which children usually develop mild seizures and then gradually lose language, first the understanding of language and later speech production ... The natural history of this condition is grim. Many of these children do not recover speech for years. Many of them became mildly to moderately mentally retarded ... No successful treatment has been adequately documented or consistently recommended.

L-carnitine: Made in muscle and liver tissue and found in certain foods, such as meat, poultry, fish, and some dairy products. It is used by many cells in the body to make energy from fat. Also called acetyl-L-carnitine hydrochloride and ALCAR.

leaky gut: Tight junctions in the gut, which control what passes through the lining of the small intestine, don't work properly and substances can leak into the bloodstream. People with celiac disease and Crohn's disease experience this. Little is known about other causes of leaky gut that aren't linked to certain types of drugs, radiation therapy, or food allergies. Leaky gut symptoms aren't unique. They're shared by other problems too. And tests often fail to uncover a definite cause of the problem. That can leave people without a diagnosis and, therefore, untreated.

Lennox-Gastaut: One of the most malignant forms of epilepsy that can be diagnosed. The syndrome usually begins between the ages of two and six, often in children who previously had infantile spasms ... Children with these multiple, difficult-to-control seizures often are given several simultaneous medications with consequent drug toxicity. The handicapping nature of the seizures, plus the drug toxicity and the continuous electrical abnormalities on the EEG, often reinforce the intrinsic brain dysfunction and produce a severely handicapped child.

lipoic acid: A type of antioxidant and chemoprotective agent. Alpha-lipoic acid is made by the body and can be found in foods such as organ meats, spinach, broccoli, peas, Brussels sprouts, and rice bran. It can also be made in the laboratory.

mercury: A silver-white, poisonous metal that is a liquid at ordinary temperatures. It is commonly used in thermometers and amalgams and has been used as an ingredient in some homeopathic medicines and in very small amounts as a preservative in viral vaccines.

magnetic resonance imaging (MRI): A procedure in which radio waves and a powerful magnet linked to a computer are used to create detailed pictures of areas inside the body. These pictures can show the difference between normal and diseased tissue. MRI makes better images of organs and soft tissue than other scanning techniques, such as computed tomography (CT) or x-ray. MRI is especially useful for imaging the brain, the spine, the soft tissue of joints, and the inside of bones.

myoclonic seizures: Jerks or twitches of the upper body, arms, or legs.

neurologist: A doctor who has special training in diagnosing and treating disorders of the nervous system.

neurotransmitter: A chemical that is released from a nerve cell, which thereby transmits an impulse from a nerve cell to another nerve, muscle, organ, or other tissue. A neurotransmitter is a messenger of neurologic information from one cell to another.

omega-3 fatty acid: A group of polyunsaturated fatty acids that are important for a number of functions in the body. The omega-3 fatty acids EPA and DHA are found in seafood, such as fatty fish (e.g., salmon, tuna, and trout) and shellfish (e.g., crab, mussels, and oysters). DHA plays important roles in the functioning of the brain and the eye. Omega-3 fatty acids may also work by decreasing the amount of triglycerides and other fats made in the liver. A different kind of omega-3, called ALA, is found in other foods, including some vegetable oils (e.g., canola and soy).

oxidative stress: A process, caused by free radicals, that can trigger cell damage. Oxidative stress is thought to play a role in a variety of diseases, including cancer, cardiovascular diseases, diabetes, Alzheimer's disease, Parkinson's disease, and eye diseases such as cataracts and age-related macular degeneration.

P-5-P: An enzyme that plays an important role in ribose (a type of sugar made in the body from glucose) metabolism.

permeable intestine: See "leaky gut."

pervasive developmental disorder (PDD): Not a term that doctors use anymore. PDDs are now called autism spectrum disorder. The name change came in 2013, when the American Psychiatric Association reclassified autistic disorder, Asperger's syndrome, childhood disintegrative disorder, and pervasive developmental disorder not otherwise specified (PDD-NOS) as autism spectrum disorders.

phenylalanine: An essential amino acid found in foods that contain protein.

primary generalized seizures: A result of abnormal neuronal activity that rapidly emerges on both sides of the brain. These seizures may cause loss of consciousness, falls, or a muscle's massive contractions.

R-5-P: The coenzyme form of vitamin B6. It can be found in certain foods such as cereals, beans, vegetables, liver, meat, and eggs. It can also be made in a laboratory. Vitamin B6 is also used for Alzheimer's disease and other types of dementia or memory loss, attention deficit hyperactivity disorder (ADHD), Down syndrome, autism, diabetes and related nerve pain, sickle cell anemia, migraine headaches, asthma, carpal tunnel syndrome, night leg cramps, muscle cramps, arthritis, preventing fractures in people with weak bones, allergies, acne and various other skin conditions, and infertility. It is also used for dizziness, motion sickness, preventing the eye disease age-related macular degeneration (AMD), seizures, convulsions due to fever, and movement disorders (tardive dyskinesia, hyperkinesis, chorea), as well as for increasing appetite and helping people remember dreams.

seizure: Seizures are symptoms of a brain problem. They happen because of sudden, abnormal electrical activity in the brain. When people think of seizures, they often think of convulsions in which a person's body shakes rapidly and uncontrollably. Not all seizures cause convulsions. There are many types of seizures, and some have mild symptoms. Seizures fall into two main groups. Focal seizures, also called partial seizures, happen in just one part of the brain. Generalized seizures are a result of abnormal activity on both sides of the brain. Most seizures last from thirty seconds to two minutes and do not cause lasting harm. However, it is a medical emergency if seizures last longer than five minutes or if a person has many seizures and does not wake up between them. Seizures can have many causes, including medicines, high fevers, head injuries, and certain diseases. People who have recurring seizures due to a brain disorder have epilepsy.

Specific Carbohydrate Diet (SCD): A strict grain-free, lactose-free, and sucrose-free dietary regimen intended for those suffering from Crohn's disease, ulcerative colitis, celiac disease, IBD, and IBS. The diet is based on the principle that specifically selected carbohydrates requiring minimal digestion are well absorbed, leaving virtually nothing for intestinal microbes to feed on.

synapse: A tiny gap between the ends of nerve fibers across which nerve impulses pass from one neuron to another; at the synapse, an impulse causes the release of a neurotransmitter, which diffuses across the gap and triggers an electrical impulse in the next neuron.

thimerosal: Thimerosal is an ethyl mercury-based preservative used in vials that contain more than one dose of a vaccine (multidose vials) to prevent germs, bacteria, and/or fungi from contaminating the vaccine.

titer: A measurement of the concentration of antibodies to a particular antigen in a blood sample. In other words, a blood test to make sure a vaccine continues to provide immunity to a particular illness.

tyrosine: The amino acid from which dopamine is made. Tyrosine is classified as a nonessential amino acid produced inside the body from phenylalanine ... Tyrosine supports and assists neurotransmitters in the brain.

ulcerative colitis (UC): A disease that causes inflammation and sores, called ulcers, in the lining of the rectum and colon. It is one of a group of diseases called inflammatory bowel disease. UC can happen at any age, but it usually starts between the ages of fifteen and thirty. It tends to run in families. The most common symptoms are pain in the abdomen and blood or pus in diarrhea.

RESOURCES AND
REFERENCES

· · · · · · · · · · · ·

Arranga, Teri (ed.), Claire I. Viadro (ed.), Lauren Underwood (ed.), and Martha Herbert (foreword). *Bugs, Bowels, and Behavior: The Groundbreaking Story of the Gut-Brain Connection.* New York: Skyhorse Publishing, 2013.

Axe, Josh. *Eat Dirt: Why Leaky Gut May Be the Root Cause of Your Health Problems and 5 Surprising Steps to Cure it.* New York: Harper Wave, 2016.

Baker, Sidney MacDonald. *Detoxification and Healing: The Key to Optimal Health.* New York: McGraw-Hill, 2003.

Barkley, Russell A. *Taking Charge of ADHD: The Complete, Authoritative Guide for Parents.* New York: Guilford Press, 2013.

Baskin, Amy, and Heather Fawcett. *More Than A Mom: Living a Full and Balanced Life When Your Child Has Special Needs.* Bethesda, MD: Woodbine House, 2006.

Batshaw, Mark L. *Children with Disabilities.* 5th ed. Baltimore: Paul H. Brookes Publishing, 2002.

Beck, Martha. *Expecting Adam.* New York: Three Rivers Press, 1999.

Bellis, Teri James. *When the Brain Can't Hear.* New York: ATRIA Books, 2002.

Bock, Kenneth and Cameron Stauth. *Healing the New Childhood Epidemics, Autism, ADHD, Asthma, and Allergies.* New York: Ballantine Books, 2007.

Bradley, Lorna. *Special Needs Parenting: From Coping to Thriving.* Minneapolis, MN: Huff Publishing Associates, 2015.

Brazelton, T. Berry. *Touchpoints, The Essential Reference: Your Child's Emotional and Behavioral Development.* Reading, MA: Perseus Books, 1992.

Brown, Brene. *The Gifts of Imperfection: Let Go of Who You Think You're Supposed to Be and Embrace Who You Are, Your Guide to a Wholehearted Life.* Center City, MN: Hazelden Publishing, 2010.

Campbell-McBride, Natasha. *Gut and Psychology Syndrome.* Cambridge, UK: Medinform Publishing, 2004.

Clinton, Hillary Rodham. *It Takes a Village: And Other Lessons Children Teach Us.* New York: Touchstone, Simon and Schuster, 1996.

Compart, Pamela J. and Dana Godbout Laake. *The Kid-Friendly ADHD and Autism Cookbook: The Ultimate Guide to the Gluten-Free, Casein-Free Diet.* Gloucester, MA: Fair Winds Press, 2009.

Conroy, Helen (Collected by) and Lisa Joyce Goes (Collected by). *The Thinking Mom's Revolution, Autism Beyond the Spectrum: Inspiring True Stories from Parents Fighting to Rescue Their Children.* New York: Skyhorse Publishing, 2013.

Crook, William G. *The Yeast Connection Handbook.* Jackson, TN: Professional Books, 2002.

Davis, William. *Wheat Belly.* New York: Rodale, 2014.

Dyer, Wayne W. *What Do You Really Want for Your Children?* New York: HarperCollins, 1985.

Eden, Donna and David Feinstein. *Energy Medicine.* New York: Penguin Putnam, 1998.

Frazier, Jan. *When Fear Falls Away, the Story of a Sudden Awakening.* San Francisco: Weiser Books, 2007.

Freeman, John M., Jennifer B. Freeman, and Millicent T. Kelly. *The Ketogenic Diet, A Treatment for Epilepsy.* New York: Demos Medical Publishing, 2000.

Freeman, John M., Eileen P. G. Vining, and Diana J. Pillas. *Seizures and Epilepsy in Childhood.* 3rd ed. Baltimore: The Johns Hopkins University Press, 2002.

Galinsky, Ellen. *Mind in The Making: The Seven Essential Life Skills Every Child Needs.* New York: Harperstudio, 2010.

Gallagher, Gina and Patricia Konjoian. *Shut Up About Your Perfect Kid: A Survival Guide for Ordinary Parents for Special Children.* New York: Three Rivers Press, 2010.

Gaulin, Cindy. *Language Processing Problems, A Guide for Parents and Teachers*. U.S.: Xlibris Corporation, 2000.

Goldberg, Michael J. with Elyse Goldberg. *The Myth of Autism: How a Misunderstood Epidemic is Destroying our Children*. New York: Skyhorse Publishing 2014.

Gottschall, Elaine. *Breaking the Vicious Cycle: Intestinal Health Through Diet*. Ontario: Kirkton Press, 2004

Hay, Louise L. *You Can Heal Your Life*. Carlsbad, CA: Hay House, 1999.

Hay, Louise L. and David Kessler. *You Can Heal Your Heart: Finding Peace After a Breakup, Divorce, or Death*. Carlsbad, CA: Hay House, 2014.

Jepson, Bryan with Jane Johnson. *Changing the Course of Autism: A Scientific Approach for Parents and Physicians*. Boulder, CO: Sentient Publications, 2007.

Kenison, Katrina. *Mitton Strings for God: Reflections for Mothers in a Hurry*. New York: Grand Central Publishing, 2000.

Kenison, Katrina. *The Gift of an Ordinary Day: A Mother's Memoir*. New York: Grand Central Publishing, 2009.

Kranowitz, Carol Stock. *The Out-of-Sync Child, Recognizing and Coping with Sensory Integration Dysfunction*. New York: Skylight Press, 1998.

Kubler-Ross, Elisabeth. *On Death and Dying: What the Dying Have to Teach Doctors, Nurses, Clergy & Their Own Families*. New York: Scribner, 1969.

Kubler-Ross, Elisabeth and David Kessler. *On Grief and Grieving: Finding the Meaning of Grief Through the Five Stages of Loss.* New York: Scribner, 2005.

Laake, Dana Godbout and Pamela J. Compart. *The ADHD and Autism Nutritional Supplement Handbook: The Cutting-Edge Biomedical Approach to Treating the Underlying Deficiencies and Symptoms of ADHD and Autism.* 3rd ed. Gloucester, MA: Fair Winds Press, 2020.

Landa, Rebecca, Mary Beth Marsden, Nancy Burrows, and Amy Newmark. *Chicken Soup for the Soul: Raising Kids on the Spectrum, 101 Inspirational Stories for Parents of Children with Autism and Asperger's.* Cos Cob, CT: Chicken Soup for the Soul Publishing, 2013.

Lewis, Lisa S. *Special Diets for Special Kids: Understanding and Implementing a Gluten and Casein Free Diet to Aid in the Treatment of Autism and Related Developmental Disorders.* Arlington, TX: Future Horizons, 1998.

Lindbergh, Anne Morrow. *Gift from the Sea.* 50th Anniversary ed. New York: Pantheon Books, 2005.

Lythcott-Haims, Julie. *How to Raise an Adult: Break Free of the Overparenting Trap and Prepare Your Kid for Success.* New York: St. Martin's Press, 2015.

Maitland, Theresa E. Laurie and Patricia O. Quinn. *Ready for Take-Off: Preparing Your Teen with ADHD or LD for College.* Washington, DC: Magination Press, 2011.

Manastra, Vincent J. *Parenting Children With ADHD: 10 Lessons That Medicine Cannot Teach.* Washington, DC: American Psychological Association Life Tools, 2014.

Marner, Kay (ed.) and Adrienne Ehlert Bashista (ed.). *Easy to Love but Hard to Raise: Real Parents, Challenging Kids, True Stories.* Pittsboro, NC: DRT Press, 2012.

Marshak, Laura E. and Fran Pollock Prezant. *Married with Special-Needs Children: A Couples' Guide to Keeping Connected.* Bethesda, MD: Woodbine House, 2007.

McCandless, Jaquelyn. *Children with Starving Brains: A Medical Treatment Guide for Autism Spectrum Disorder.* 4th ed. Wilton Manors, FL: Bramble Books, 2009.

McCarthy, Jenny. *Mother Warriors: A Nation of Parents Healing Autism Against All Odds.* New York: Plume, 2009.

Meyer, Donald (ed.). *Thicker than Water: Essays by Adult Siblings of People with Disabilities.* Bethesda, MD: Woodbine House, 2009.

Meyer, Donald (ed.). *Views from Our Shoes: Growing Up with a Brother or Sister with Special Needs.* Bethesda, MD: Woodbine House, 1997.

Minocha, Anil. *Is It Leaky Gut or Leaky Gut Syndrome?* Shreveport, LA: LOGOS Enterprises LLC, 2014.

Moore, Thomas. *Care of the Soul.* New York: HarperCollins, 1992.

Neurological Health. https://neurologicalhealth.org

Philo, Jolene. *Different Dream Parenting: A Practical Guide to Raising a Child with Special Needs.* Grand Rapids, MI: Discovery House, 2011.

Quinn, Patricia O. (ed.). *ADD and the College Student: A Guide for High School and College Students with Attention Deficit Disorder.* Washington, D.C.: Magination Press, 2001.

Rapp, Doris. *Is This Your Child? Discovering and Treating Unrecognized Allergies in Children and Adults.* New York: William Morrow and Company, 1991.

Richardson, Cheryl. *The Art of Extreme Self-Care.* Carlsbad, CA: Hay House, Inc. 2009

Robison, John Elder. *Be Different: Adventures of a Free-Range Aspergian, With Practical Advice for Aspergians, Misfits, Families, and Teachers.* New York: Crown Archetype, 2011.

Robison, John Elder. *Look Me in The Eye: My Life with Asperger's.* New York: Broadway Paperbacks, 2008.

Rotbart, Harley A. *No Regrets Parenting: Turning Long Days and Short Years into Cherished Moments with Your Kids.* Kansas City, MO: Andrews McMeel Publishing, 2012.

Ruiz, Don Miguel. *The Mastery of Love.* San Rafael, CA: Amber-Allen Publishing, 1999.

Sarkis, Stephanie Moulton. *Making the Grade with A+DD: A Student's Guide to Succeeding in College with Attention Deficit Disorder.* Oakland, CA: New Harbinger Publication, 2008.

Schor, Edward L. (ed. in chief). *The American Academy of Pediatrics, Caring for Your School-Age Child, Ages 5 to 12, The Complete and Authoritative Guide.* New York: Bantam Books, 1995.

Seroussi, Karyn. *Unraveling the Mystery of Autism and Pervasive Developmental Disorder.* New York: Simon & Schuster, 2000.

Seuss, Dr. *Horton Hears a Who.* New York: Random House, 1954.

Shaw, William. *Biological Treatments for Autism & PDD: Causes and Biomedical Therapies for Autism and PDD.* U.S.: William Shaw, PhD, 2008.

Shaw, William. *Autism Beyond the Basics: Treating Autism Spectrum Disorders.* U.S.:William Shaw, PhD, 2009.

Shelov, Steven P. (ed. in chief), and Robert E. Hannemann (assoc. medical ed.). *The American Academy of Pediatrics, The Complete and Authoritative Guide, Caring for Your Baby and Young Child, Birth to Age 5.* New York: Bantam Books, 1998.

Singer, Jonathan. *The Special Needs Parent Handbook: Critical Strategies and Practical Advice to Help You Survive and Thrive.* Tenafly, NJ: Clinton+Valley Publishing, 2012.

Solomon, Andrew. *Far from the Tree: Parents, Children, and the Search for Identity.* New York: Scribner, 2012.

Stixrud, William and Ned Johnson. *The Self-Driven Child: The Science and Sense of Giving Your Kids More Control Over Their Lives.* New York: Viking, 2018.

Strohm, Kate. *Being the Other One: Growing Up with a Brother or Sister Who Has Special Needs.* Boston: Shambhala Publications, 2005.

The Autism Exchange. www.theautismexchange.com

Williamson, Marianne. *A Return to Love: Reflections on the Principles of a Course in Miracles.* New York: HarperCollins, 1992.

ENDNOTES

. . . .

Chapter 1

[1] "Types of Seizures," Epilepsy Foundation, accessed January 22, 2019, www.epilepsy.com/learn/types-seizures.

Chapter 2

[1] "About IDEA," Individuals with Disabilities Education Act, accessed January 29, 2019, www.sites.ed.gov/idea/about-idea.

[2] John M. Freeman, Eileen P. G. Vining, and Diana J. Pillas, *Seizures and Epilepsy in Childhood,* 3rd ed. (Baltimore: The Johns Hopkins University Press, 2002), 122.

[3] Freeman, Vining, and Pillas. *Seizures and Epilepsy in Childhood,* 121.

[4] "Healthy Lifestyle," Adult Health, Mayo Clinic, accessed January 22, 2019, www.mayoclinic.org/healthy-lifestyle/adult-health/in-depth/denial/art-20047926.

[5] Jonathan Singer, *The Special Needs Parent Handbook: Critical Strategies and Practical Advice to Help You Survive and Thrive* (Tenafly, NJ: Clinton+Valley Publishing, 2012), 3.

[6] "Patient Care and Health Info," Mayo Clinic, accessed January 22, 2019, www.mayoclinic.org/search/search-results?q=ketogenic%20diet.

Chapter 3

[1] "Autism Spectrum Disorder, Frequently Asked Questions on Mitochondrial Disease," Centers for Disease Control, accessed January 29, 2019, www.cdc.gov/ncbddd/autism/mitochondrial-faq.html.

[2] "Environmental Factors in Autism," Autism Speaks, accessed January 31, 2019, www.autismspeaks.org/environmental-factors-autism.

[3] "Q & A on Part B of IDEA 2004: Purposes and Key Definitions," Center for Parent Information and Resources, accessed January 21, 2019, www.parentcenterhub.org/qa1/.

[4] Bill Healey, "Helping Parents Deal with the Fact That Their Child Has a Disability," LD Online, accessed January 31, 2019, www.ldonline.org/article/5937/?theme=print.

[5] "What is Autism," Autism Society, accessed February 5, 2019, www.autism-society.org/what-is/.

Chapter 4

[1] "Microbial Etiology of the GI Tract," Great Plains Laboratory, accessed November 15, 2010, www.greatplainslaboratory.com/candida-and-yeast-overgrowth/?rq=number%20of%20microorganisms%20in%20the%20GI%20tract%20.

[2] "Health, Metabolism, and Nutrition: Food Allergies, Allergy or Chemical Reaction?" Great Plains Laboratory, accessed November 17, 2010, www.gpl4u.com/food-allergy.asp.

3   "Autism and Insurance Coverage: State Laws," National Conference of State Legislators (NCSL), accessed March 5, 2019, www.ncsl.org/research/health/autism-and-insurance-coverage-state-laws.aspx.

4   Jennifer B. Saunders, "Overwhelmed by Autism: A Dramatic Increase in Diagnoses has Lawmakers Debating the State's Role," NCSL, accessed January 31, 2019, www.ncsl.org/Portals/1/Documents/magazine/articles/2010/SL_1010-Autism.pdf?ver=2010-10-05-110307-857.

5   "Federal Health Pulse, Health Wise: Reflections on World Autism Awareness Day & HHS Autism Awareness Month," NCSL Bulletin of Federal Actions, April 2, 2012, accessed January 31, 2019, www.ncsl.org/documents/statefed/health/FedHlthPul40212.pdf.

6   "About Genova Diagnostics," accessed March 5, 2019, www.facebook.com/genova.diagnostics/about/.

7   "Vitamin and Mineral Supplement Fact Sheets," the National Institutes of Health, Office of Dietary Supplements, accessed January 29, 2019, www.ods.od.nih.gov/factsheets/list-VitaminsMinerals/.

Chapter 5

1   William Shaw, "Yeast Overgrowth, The Yeast Problem and Bacteria Byproducts: Summary," the Great Plains Laboratory, accessed January 31, 2019, www.gpl4u.com/italian/yeast2.html#giecology.

2 "Breaking the Cycle of ADHD," Great Plains Laboratory, accessed November 15, 2010, www.greatplainslaboratory.com/search?q=breaking%20the%20cycle.

3 Natasha Campbell-McBride, *Gut and Psychology Syndrome* (Cambridge, UK: Medinform, 2004), 60.

Chapter 6

1 "Carcinoid Syndrome," Patient Care & Health Info., Mayo Clinic, accessed February 22, 2019, www.mayoclinic.org/diseases-conditions/carcinoid-syndrome/symptoms-causes/syc-20370666.

2 Kate Strohm, *Being the Other One: Growing Up with a Brother or Sister Who Has Special Needs* (Boston: Shambhala, 2005), 31.

3 Strohm, *Being the Other One: Growing Up with a Brother or Sister Who Has Special Needs, xiii.*

Chapter 7

1 Laura Marshak and Fran Pollock Prezant, Married with Special-Needs Children: A Couples' Guide to Keeping Connected, (Bethesda, MD: Woodbine House, 2007), viii.

2 Marshak and Prezant, *Married with Special-Needs Children: A Couples' Guide to Keeping Connected,* 12.

3 Strohm, *Being the Other One: Growing Up with a Brother or Sister Who Has Special Needs,* 131.

Chapter 8

[1] "About NCRC Pre School," National Child Research Center, accessed February 5, 2019, www.ncrcpreschool.org/about-ncrc.

[2] "Curriculum," National Child Research Center, accessed March 11, 2019, www.ncrcpreschool.org/curriculum/inclusion.

[3] Elisabeth Kubler-Ross and David Kessler, *On Grief and Grieving: Finding the Meaning of Grief Through the Five Stages of Loss,* (New York, Scribner, 2005), 29.

[4] Kubler-Ross and Kessler, *On Grief and Grieving: Finding the Meaning of Grief Through the Five Stages of Loss,* 31.

Chapter 9

[1] "About Dana Laake Nutrition," accessed November 15, 2010, www.DanaLaake.com. Current contact, www.facebook.com/Dana-Laake-Nutrition-118506546774/

[2] "Health Care, Lifetime and Annual Limits," US Department of Health and Human Services, accessed March 8, 2019, www.hhs.gov/healthcare/about-the-aca/benefit-limits/index.html.

Chapter 10

[1] Kubler-Ross and David Kessler, On Grief and Grieving: Finding the Meaning of Grief Through the Five Stages of Loss, 33-34.

2   Marshak and Prezant, *Married with Special-Needs Children: A Couples' Guide to Keeping Connected*, 3-6.

3   Jan Frazier, *When Fear Falls Away: The Story of a Sudden Awakening*, (San Francisco, RedWheel/Weiser Books, 2007), 81.

Chapter 11

1   "What is Neuropsychology," accessed November 15, 2010, www.nanonline.org.

2   Lorna Bradley, *Special Needs Parenting: From Coping to Thriving*, (Minneapolis: Huff Publishing, 2015), 9.

3   Bradley, *Special Needs Parenting: From Coping to Thriving*, 18.

4   Bradley, *Special Needs Parenting: From Coping to Thriving*, 17.

5   "The Neuropsychological Evaluation," The Stixrud Group, accessed November 20, 2010, www.stixrud.com.

Chapter 12

1   Strohm, Being the Other One: Growing Up with a Brother or Sister Who Has Special Needs, 45.

\ information can be obtained
w.ICGtesting.com
in the USA
032040061020
BV00001B/6

Chapter 13

1 Kubler-Ross and Kessler, On Grief and Grieving: Finding the Meaning of Grief Through the Five Stages of Loss, 33-37.

2 Campbell-McBride, *Gut and Psychology Syndrome,* 53.

3 Campbell-McBride, *Gut and Psychology Syndrome,* 57.

4 Campbell-McBride, *Gut and Psychology Syndrome,*6-7.

Chapter 14

1 Michael Goldberg with Elyse Goldberg, The Myth of Autism: How a Misunderstood Epidemic is Destroying ou' Children, (New York: Skyhorse Publishing, 2014), 144.

2 "Cognitive-Behavioral Therapy," Children and Adult' Attention Deficit Disorder (CHADD), accessed March www.chadd.org/for-adults/cognitive-behavioral-tl'

3 Theresa E. Laurie Maitland, and Patricia O. C *for Take-Off: Preparing Your Teen With AI College*, (Washington, DC: Magination Pre

4 Katrina Kenison, *The Gift of an Ordin* *Memoir*, (New York: Grand Central ᵀ

5 MedlinePlus, the National Institu' Library of Medicine, acces' medlineplus.gov.